PRAISE FOR *IT'S YOUR BIRTH... RIGHT?*

"I recently read *It's Your Birth... Right?* and Cherie Pasion's passion clearly shines through. Cherie wonderfully and gently guides new parents to a calmer and happier place. I loved the way she guided me to connect with the new me, and led me to a stronger connection with my new bundle of joy and also with those around me—I would definitely recommend this book to my friends who are expecting a baby."

Kirstie Stockx, Author of *Self Care for New Mums*

"I find this book to be a valuable resource for modern women expecting their first child, or going through pregnancy again after a long gap. We need all the reminders we can get—in the masculine society working women often find themselves in—that our femininity and our natural strengths and tendencies are powerful and worth cherishing and developing. A great gift for every professional mother-to-be."

Emily M Morgan, Author and Director, Parent Resource Centre

"A heart-felt read that took me on a journey of self-discovery and deepened my understanding of the 'new' me as a mother, strengthening my relationship with my daughter. This is not a survival guide to parenting, but rather a tool to break down the boundaries and build deep emotional connections with your child, yourself and your family. I recommend this book for all new mums and mums-to-be."

Allison Muller, Director, Big Wave Ventures

"Cherie is passionate about helping professional women transition into parenthood. Having swapped stories about our pregnancy/birthing/parenting history it is clear Cherie has an unwavering commitment to women having what they need to engage in an honest and open discussion both within themselves and those they love about how they are faring and preparing through what can be a tumultuous time. Cherie's commitment to honouring her own process has infused this warm, informative and practical nurturing book. As a professional woman becoming a mother for the first time I could have really d̶̶̶̶̶̶̶̶̶̶̶

Dr Linda Wilson, *...eling Women Off The Ceiling*

T0163749

It's Your Birth... Right?

IT'S YOUR BIRTH...RIGHT?

A Guide for Professional Women to
Calmly Transition to Motherhood

CHERIE PASION

NEW YORK

NASHVILLE • MELBOURNE • VANCOUVER

It's Your Birth... Right?

A Guide for Professional Women to Calmly Transition to Motherhood

Published in New York, New York, by Morgan James Publishing. Morgan James is a trademark of Morgan James, LLC. www.MorganJamesPublishing.com

The Morgan James Speakers Group can bring authors to your live event. For more information or to book an event visit The Morgan James Speakers Group at www.TheMorganJamesSpeakersGroup.com.

ISBN 9781683503774 paperback
ISBN 9781683503781 Ebook
Library of Congress Control Number: 2016919689

Cover Design by:
Ryan McDonald-Smith
www.youniquecreation.com and

Megan Whitney
megan@creativeninjadesigns.com

Interior Design by:
Simon Rattray
www.squirtcreative.com and

Chris Treccani
www.3dogdesign.net

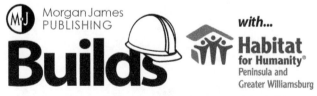

In an effort to support local communities, raise awareness and funds, Morgan James Publishing donates a percentage of all book sales for the life of each book to Habitat for Humanity Peninsula and Greater Williamsburg.

Get involved today! Visit
www.MorganJamesBuilds.com

CONTENT PAGE

ACKNOWLEDGEMENTS

A book isn't the effort of one person—it is the work of many. I'd like to bring to light the wonderful contributions made to this book by others and thank those who supported the process along the way.

To my wonderful husband Leland, with whom I'm privileged to walk in life's adventure, and our son, Juan, who softened my masculine heart and showed me that connections are everything. Thank you for your patience, love and support.

To my parents and parents-in-laws, brothers and sisters, nieces and nephews—thank you for the love and support and the wonderful family bond we share.

To Megan Malone and the team at Morgan James Publishing— thank you for your wonderful support. To Jacqui Pretty and Carolyn Jackson at Grammar Factory. Jacqui—thank you for the support and opportunities. Carolyn—my goodness, you are an angel and a magician. Your gentle but firm touch with this book was astounding.

To the contributors to this book—Annette Baulch from OzTantra and Kathleen Marcoux from Tree of Life Yoga—thank you for the efforts and insight you selflessly shared.

To Amanda Bigelow—thank you. I am deeply appreciative of the support, encouragement and friendship we have developed through our book writing journey.

To my mentors, Andrew Griffiths, Chris Knight and Luna Wood— words cannot adequately express the gratitude and respect I have for you.

To Melissa Spilsted, who first opened my eyes that birth and becoming a mother can be calm and empowering. Thank you, you did much more than help me have a positive birth experience, you changed the course of my life.

To my many friends, thank you for all of your love and support.

To the readers of this book, I also want to thank you for trusting me with your precious transition to motherhood.

INTRODUCTION

Every time a baby is born, so too is a mother.

You watch the second line develop on your pregnancy test, hardly daring to believe the results. If you're like me, there's a back-up test ready. It too shows the second line appearing and reality sinks in. You're going to be a mother. In that moment, everything changes.

The awakening to motherhood happens in that moment. There is a stirring and opening in your heart—of new possibilities, of planning for your future. What follows is a journey of emotions as you understand the enormity of the coming changes. The elation and excitement are mixed with fear and doubts.

I've written this book for you to use as an accompaniment in your journey to motherhood, to help guide you in the tender business of emotional preparation.

I remember when I found out I was pregnant. I was more fearful than excited. I had a great career flying around the country implementing business technology solutions and I didn't know if I was ready for that to change. Yet, I could feel something shift within my heart and I knew this new experience of motherhood was exactly the growth and development I needed.

I searched for materials to help me emotionally in this growth and evolution into my future self and to help me see how I could set my family up for the best start possible, but I wasn't able to find the materials I was looking for in one place.

So I was inspired to create this book to help you birth not only your baby, but also who you are as a mother as you step temporarily or permanently outside of your career to have and raise your newborn baby.

Many materials related to the motherhood transition are birth and baby-centric. This book is mother-centric. It's about setting up a series of connections that will not only help you stay strong and resilient, but will also introduce a softness that is crucial to a healthy transition. This book will not attempt to control what cannot be controlled. While it will help you clarify what you would like to happen in your transition to motherhood, a key concept it teaches is that of letting go and accepting outcomes that cannot be changed.

This book will not replace medical advice. While many of the concepts in this book are not mainstream—you could even call some of them 'new age'—they're not meant to be an alternative to the incredible expertise offered by the medical establishment. They're intended as a *complement* to traditional medical care.

You will, however, as a result of reading this book and following the practical examples, walk away with a sense of empowerment in this pivotal time of your life. It will give you a compass to follow throughout your pregnancy, the birth of your child and the early months of motherhood. These three stages of your transition are visited in each step of the compass, so you may wish to revisit the book as you reach different stages and milestones in your journey.

This book is an invitation to form deep connections starting from within.

PART 1:

CONNECTIONS ARE THE HEART OF MOTHERHOOD

'If you've ever wondered why new parents are so unbearable to be around, it's because they are overwhelmed by the strength of their personal transformation.'

STEPHEN MARCHE

Childbearing is the most natural thing in the world. The oldest human remains have been dated at 195,000 years and for each of us to even be in this world, 16,000 people had to procreate in the last 400 years.[1] But while the biology of conception, pregnancy and childbirth has not changed in that time, the role that women play in society has.

IMPORTANCE OF EMOTIONAL PREPARATION

It is only in the recent past that many women have stepped out of their traditional, confined roles of nurturer, nester and mother and taken on new roles such as income-earner, power-broker and society-leader. While there have always been mothers who also worked or made their mark on society, the phenomenon of the working mother has only recently become commonplace. Now is a time when women who define themselves primarily as professionals are also becoming mothers. This new type of woman faces a set of challenges that are quite different from those of previous generations' experience of motherhood.

Struggling to cope emotionally

I first noticed that professional women were finding the transition to motherhood emotionally challenging shortly after becoming a mother myself. While I experienced my fair share of anxious moments, I felt reasonably comfortable in my new role. Yet through the new motherhood fog I saw that my peers—other highly intelligent, strong women in various professions—were struggling to cope in their new role.

Research by Dr Bronwyn Harman at Edith Cowan University has shown that professional women, in particular, have a tough time transitioning to motherhood. In her interviews with thousands

3

of women, she has consistently found that the realities of early motherhood didn't live up to their anticipations. This was particularly true for women who had enjoyed a successful professional career, and were accustomed to control, predictability and productivity. Upon becoming mothers, they experienced a strong feeling of loss (of identity and power), isolation and fatigue.[2]

In the early days of my motherhood experience, I experienced this to some degree and witnessed it among my peers and in sentiments in parenting blogs, online and print magazines. I remember once when asked how I was coping and I tentatively admitted motherhood was proving easier than I expected, I was scoffed at.

I was surprised by this. I wasn't fundamentally any different from other mothers. I wasn't particularly special. I wouldn't describe my innate nature as calm and I'm certainly not unflappable.

So why was my motherhood transition calm?

Before understanding the answer lay in finding connections and preparing emotionally, over the next two years I reflected deeply on this question. I researched. I joined groups to understand the everyday fears, anxieties and challenges that expectant and new mothers face. I talked with pregnant women and mothers, with energy healers, with people who had walked a path similar to mine and with people who had walked a different one. I devoured books and article after article. I also looked back into the history of childbirth and early motherhood to understand how it has evolved over time.

After much research, I discovered a couple of key themes that influence how we prepare emotionally. The first theme relates to commonly held beliefs. The second theme relates to an imbalance in our core energy.

Uncovering beliefs

During my research a number of beliefs relating to the transition to motherhood kept rising to the surface, particularly when looking at perceptions that professional women have. Many of these beliefs were uncovered after women had their children and were reflecting on their ideals and thoughts coming into motherhood.

The commonly held beliefs are:
- Parenting is a matter of winging it. As babies don't come with an instruction manual, there is little point preparing for when baby arrives.
- Of the preparations taken, they are baby-centric, physical and material in nature.
- Childbirth is something to get through or be endured for a positive reward at the end.
- The same approach for career success can be used for success in having and raising a child.
- Identity is tightly associated with our professions.
- It's a sign of weakness to ask for help.

These commonly-held beliefs unfortunately are holding women back from having a cool-headed, calm and connected transition to motherhood. Underpinning each of those beliefs is a lack of mother-centric emotional and mental preparation for this period of change. This means that foundations are often shaken when bub arrives and feelings become elevated. The highs are pronounced but women also face anxiety, a great deal of uncertainty and even depression.

The good news is that beliefs can be changed. As you're exposed to new information and create connections, the neural pathways in your brain can be rewired to form a new set of beliefs that better suits your circumstances and the journey you wish to take.

It's *your* birth experience, right? So take control and say goodbye to beliefs that no longer serve you. Throughout this book you will find knowledge and activities that will help you do this.

Balancing your two core energies

Another underlying theme I uncovered was an imbalance in the core energies running through our bodies. Let me explain.

We are all comprised of both masculine and feminine energies. Feminine energy embodies qualities of creation, nurturing, intuition and being. Masculine energy embodies qualities such as logic, willpower, planning and action. The concept of yin and yang is an expression of these two complementary energies. Before I became pregnant I was aware of yin and yang, but had written it off as some hippy mumbo-jumbo. But after I became pregnant I discovered the strength of being centred in yin and yang and just how crucial it is during pregnancy and early motherhood.

During my pregnancy I felt a discord with the conventional path—the masculine path—I was being led down. I understood it was important to have blood tests and scans and book into hospitals and consult obstetricians, but my intuition was yearning for more. My intuition was telling me to find mentors who could help me grow and evolve as a woman and as a mother. To spend time in nature and in water. To slow down and enjoy the feeling of being pregnant. To enjoy the bond between my son and I—to lose myself in it. To connect deeply with my husband. To look inwards and assess my own beliefs, fears and expectations. I didn't realise then that I was actually bringing my feminine energy forward and in balance with the masculine.

It will come as no surprise that, as professional women, we have become marvellously adept at over-engaging our masculine energy. Women have developed masculine shells as we have built our careers, taken a major role in managing our household and finances, and shared our gifts with the world. As professionals, we're used to being in our heads—we're used to being in control, strategising, analysing and doing. This isn't necessarily a bad thing; I, for one, am proud of all I have achieved and thankful that I grew up in an era that supported this independence.

But motherhood is a time of transformation guided by feminine energy. Gestating a baby, giving birth and nurturing a baby is a creative process that requires us to step into our feminine energy and be fully aware of what's happening in our bodies. Becoming a mother is a time when we need to allow ourselves to listen to our heart, intuition and instincts more than any other time in our lives. And here is where the trouble lies.

When entering motherhood, a majority of professional women are still operating with a masculine energy bias—we are trying to use the same methods we used in our careers to have and raise our babies. It's not our fault. In today's masculine-based society, we haven't been given a roadmap to indicate how to engage with our feminine energy and fully listen to our intuition. This means that the transition to motherhood can be a time of disconnection. For many women, feelings of fear and anxiety, identity loss and uncertainty come to the surface. These feelings serve to disempower women who are used to operating from a place of power and control.

Thankfully, using the tools and techniques in this book, you will be able to find a roadmap to connect with your feminine energy.

The importance of finding balance

The key to finding your personal power is to find balance in the yin and yang—to find the centre. Take the opposing qualities of strength and weakness, for example. You may be thinking, 'If there is a choice, I'll go strength any day.' But here's the thing, weakness is the opposite of strength, so it has equal potency. I'm sure you know what happens when you're constantly strong. At some point you burn out. Your body becomes ill and you start feeling weak. The aim is to be centred— to have a balance between the two qualities. Where weakness meets strength in relatively equal measure, there is harmony and health.

It's similar with the ups and downs of motherhood, the balance is the centre of your masculine and feminine energies. Both energies have equal potency. So it's important to utilise your well-honed skills of connecting with the masculine, but it's of equal importance to learn how to embrace your feminine energy.

I don't want to set any false expectations. Transitioning to motherhood consists of ongoing change, and it can be tough to keep up. There will be difficult days, and meeting the needs of a wholly dependent baby doesn't always come naturally, but there can be a balance and you can find your centre. And from that centre, you can begin your journey into motherhood.

Connection is at the centre

Finding connections is at the heart of engaging your feminine and centring it with the masculine. Becoming a mother is really about understanding the heart of connections:

- Conceiving, gestating and giving life to your baby sets up a connection and bond that lasts a lifetime.
- Conceiving a child and creating a new life is the ultimate connection with your partner.
- Becoming a parent connects us to our own parents, whom we may now see in a different light and perhaps begin to understand a bit better.
- Pregnancy is a time to connect with your past. It's a time to heal and forgive, to celebrate and express gratitude. It allows you to sift through your past and identify what you want to contribute to the next generation.
- Parenting also connects us on a deep level with other parents— just ask any mother how they feel when they read a news story that involves a child, whether that story is heart-warming or devastating.
- Having a baby connects whole family lines. Bringing a child into the world connects you and your child to the generations that came before you and sets up a pathway for connection with generations to come.

- Having a child connects us with strangers. I didn't realise how powerful this was until I was out and about with a young baby. People would stop me in the street and want to look at my son, or ask to touch his tiny feet or fingers. They would talk about when their children were babies. It was a way for them to remember. I was deeply moved by these connections.

The ultimate connection, however, is with ourselves. The journey through conception, pregnancy and birth ultimately results in a metamorphosis—we become a mother.

THE CONNECTION COMPASS

Metaphorically, the motherhood journey is like trekking in the Himalaya. You will have days of easy and happy walking in beautiful valleys with the sun shining—thinking that each moment is the pinnacle in your journey until a few steps later when the view gets even more spectacular. Other days (or even minutes later) you will be climbing endless, uphill paths with no end in sight in cold, drenching rain—you will be challenged and fatigued, your body and mind will both be weary, and your emotions will be running high.

But, just as you would make careful preparations for a trek in the Himalaya, so you need to make careful preparations for your transition to motherhood. If you were trekking in the Himalaya, an essential part of your preparation would be to acquire a compass and learn how to use it. You need a compass so you can be sure to go in the right direction from the outset, rather than wander aimlessly and hope you're going the right way. What if you had a compass that could help you navigate the transition into motherhood?

This book gives you just that—what I call a 'connection compass' that will guide you and help you transition to motherhood from a place of personal power.

How the connection compass will help you

The transition to motherhood is a unique process for every family, as no two families come into parenthood with the same beliefs, backgrounds and circumstances. Over-simplifying the messages around entering parenthood is unhelpful. Common messages, such as 'you will instantly fall in love with your baby', 'motherhood comes intuitively', 'sleep while the baby is sleeping', 'accept all help that is offered', are well-meaning, but families need to find a groove that suits them.

The connection compass helps you to prepare for motherhood according to your own unique circumstances. There are certainly common themes and patterns that arise during the transformation to motherhood and these are discussed, but the book is focused on you tapping into your own resources and creating a journey that is uniquely yours. It allows you and your partner to step into parenthood from a place of authenticity and centredness.

Following the compass will not make you soft, weak and dependent. Feminine energy allows you to access incredible strength, and while I encourage you to tap into that energy to guide you in your motherhood journey, I also acknowledge the power of the masculine and recognise that a balance of the two is key.

The connection compass highlights four directions of preparation that will reduce your fears and anxiety and enable a pathway of empowerment:

- **CONNECT WITH YOU:** You will look inward to gain clarity, understand the essence of who you are and uncover any blockages, fears and expectations you may be bringing into your motherhood journey.
- **CONNECT WITH YOUR BABY:** You will develop the platform for deep, lifelong bonds with your child by engaging in the five senses before, during and after birth.

- **CONNECT WITH OTHERS:** You will learn how to maintain a connection with your partner and also how to create a 'village' to support you.
- **CONNECT WITH NATURE:** As nature is at the heart of feminine energy, you will learn how best to spend time in nature during this transformational period, helping you go through a healing and nurturing process.

Each connection point is described in depth followed by a chapter that describes a number of bite-sized activities you can do daily and weekly to help you maintain the connections you forge along the way.

Using your connection compass

Throughout the book you'll find several activities to complete. I recommend that you find a beautiful journal that will be your companion and confidant through this journey of discovery. Over time it's likely that new expectations, new fears and new ideas will come up and your journal can be a place to capture and release all of these insights. Later, you can look through the journal as a reminder of how far you have come.

Having a compass to follow in your journey allows you to put down roots and ground yourself during this transition period, a period unlike anything you've experienced before. It allows you to open up and connect with a solid base so you don't vacillate to and fro, out of balance, out of kilter. Instead, during difficult periods in your journey you can draw upon the point on the compass that will provide you with what you need. This enables you to be like bamboo; your strength allowing you to be flexible and bend the way the wind blows.

So let's begin.

PART 2:

CONNECT WITH YOU

'What lies behind us and what lies before us are tiny matters compared to what lies within us.'

RALPH WALDO EMERSON

There is no greater preparation you can make for your transition into motherhood than connecting with yourself. This section is about looking within. It's a deep dive into who you really are, so you can enter motherhood from a point of understanding and be able to draw on your personal power.

You need a deep connection with yourself in order to parent in a calm and confident way. Connecting with who you are will allow you to tap into a wellspring of resilience and strength that perhaps you didn't even know was there. You will be able to recognise when you're running on empty and need support. You will be open enough to ask for help. You will be in touch with your intuition. You will be able to step into parenting from the point of your own authentic self.

It's especially important to connect with yourself because there is no one-size-fits-all approach to mothering. Every single one of us comes into parenting with a different worldview, with different personal circumstances, health concerns, attitudes, expectations and experience. Be wary of any expert who tells you that their way is the only way. It was the way that helped them in their specific circumstances, with their background, expectations and experience. If you're in touch with your true self, you're more likely to know whether their advice is also right for you.

It's useful to start this personal exploration *before* you become a mother. When bub arrives and you're in the middle of chaos with raging hormones, when you're exhausted, frustrated and lonely, it will become difficult to find the time and space to do this important work.

This chapter will help you to handle change, problems and stress more effectively, and help you to trust yourself to manage your transition to motherhood.

FIND YOU

'You're not broken. You don't need fixing. You are a divine being with infinite potential and it's time to realise how magnificent you are. It's time to put yourself first and access the gift that you are right now.'–Panache Desai

Having a baby is life-changing. It is indescribable. Meeting your precious baby after being inseparably attached for the previous nine months is miraculous. When I first held my son in my arms it was almost surreal. His tiny little features—puffy eyes, squashed-up face, wrinkly fingers—made him so precious and strange and beautiful and delicate all at the same time. He traced my face and his father's face with his eyes and started licking his lips. Leland and I were absolutely besotted and in total awe.

A new little person was added to our lives. We were now a family. But with this addition, little did I know that I'd come to feel like I had lost something of myself.

Some days I questioned who I was. I knew that who I was had grown and expanded—I was now a mother to the most beautiful baby. I experienced an opening and outpouring of love that would make me burst into an eruption of tears of love and fulfilment and joy. Yet, I also felt a bit lost, even a bit aimless.

My job and all my experiences prior to being a mum didn't seem to matter to people anymore. Instead, I was this little cutie-pie's mother. I loved being a mum but I was also confused by it— who was I now?

Before having your baby, you're relatively free to do as you please, and have a sense of control over your life and are able to shape who you are. During your pregnancy, you know there will be change ahead, but you're not sure exactly how or what that will look like or what sort of impact it will have on your life. Therefore, it may not seem important at this stage to start looking deeper inwards. Some women may be wary of these changes and hold onto their identity even more tightly as they worry their employers, colleagues and clients may already see them as mothers and may question their future commitment. If this is the case, you may not *want* to look inwards.

Then, all of a sudden, your baby is born and their needs are all-encompassing. Some women say that they aren't even able to take a shower when they're at home by themselves with a new baby. I remember times when I was hungry and I'd be preparing lunch for myself while my son was sleeping or playing. Then, suddenly, he'd cry and I'd have no choice but to turn off the stove, with lunch half-cooked, having no idea when I could get back to it.

It's this lack of control over simple tasks like taking a shower or eating lunch that can make us feel like we're in the passenger seat heading to an unknown destination. And that can be really scary for a lot of us. Hence, our sense of self can diminish.

I have my own theory on losing self during the motherhood transition. I wonder whether many of us even know who we are—truly, deeply—in the first place. I wonder whether it is not so much that we lose our identity but that motherhood amplifies a disconnection of self. How many of us associate our identity to what we do, rather than who we truly are? So when our professional role is stripped back, we are left wondering what has become of us.

Eckhart Tolle, author of *The Power of Now*, has said that an essential ingredient in most kinds of suffering is a diminishment of one's sense of self. Yet, in reality, what feels like a loss of our identity is actually the crumbling of an image of who we held ourselves to be in our minds. Tolle describes that sense of self as a mental fiction.[3] It is the ego.

This is good news, because when who you *think* you are dissolves, you can start exploring who you *really* are. If you feel a sense of loss, you can celebrate it as a way to open and awaken to new possibilities of who you are. Of course, it's also possible to start this process *before* you're lost. And it will be easier to get in touch with the essence of 'you' while still pregnant, when you have more space and time for self-reflection. This saves some anxiety and doubt down the track. So while you're still in a space where you feel confident in your identity, I'd like you to do the following exercise.

\\\\\\\\\\\\\\\\\\\\ EXERCISE ////////////////////////

In doing this exercise, I want you to tap into your feminine energy to guide you. You can't think your passion and your purpose, you have to feel it. You will know when you find what reflects your authentic self; you will know it in your heart and your stomach. You will feel it.

Before you start this exercise, take several deep breaths. This will allow you to slow down and relax into the exercise. You can also follow some of the breathing exercises listed in the last section of this book.

Take out your journal and follow these self-inquiry prompts, paying attention to your emotions as you list your answers. Paying attention to your emotions will help you discover the things you particularly love. If you find yourself smiling or experience a fluttering in your stomach, you'll know you are close to your passion.

1) Remember when you were a child. What did you want to be when you grew up?

List all the options you can remember. Now ask yourself why you wanted to be those things. Dig deep to uncover the essence of what your list means.

For example, when I was young I wanted to be:
- A policewoman
- An aid worker in India
- The author of a book about Indigenous Australian culture
- A national parks ranger
- An explorer
- A palaeontologist

These roles seem so unrelated and random. Yet, when I asked myself why I wanted to do or be these things, I realised they were all about helping people, empowerment, uncovering, discovering and exploring.

2) Go for a walk around your home. Observe and write down the type of things you surround yourself with:
   - How do you decorate your house?
   - What sort of wall hangings do you have?
   - What kind of books do you have on your bookshelf?
   - Do you have a balcony or garden? What is it like?
   - What type of music do you listen to?
   - What clothes do you wear?
   - What do you keep in your car?

   Can you see any common themes? For example, do you surround yourself with artifacts from your travels, or do your possessions reflect your love of vintage, or some other defined style?

3) What do you spend your money on? You probably spend your discretionary income on things you love, like travel, fashion, books, music and hobbies.

4) Have a think about what you really love to do. Think about the different ways you spend your time and what brings you the most joy. Observe what makes you smile when you think about it. Observe how your body feels as you think about these things. List as many points as you can. Do you feel joy when you're:
   - With your partner?
   - With friends?
   - Preparing for your baby?

- By yourself?
- At work?
- At yoga?
- Travelling?
- Spending time at the beach?
- Being in nature?

5) Now go through your responses and identify any underlying themes. Prioritise into the top 2-3 themes that bring you the most joy.

\\   /////////////////////////////////////

After doing the above exercise and once you have an idea of themes or common factors running through your responses, think of ways you can integrate these aspects of your true self when you have your baby. What activities can you do when you are comfortable to go and about with your baby? Are there groups or meet-ups you can join to be connected with like-minded people?

For instance, if you love art, you could keep a colouring book for adults or a sketch pad in the pram. Or if you love reading, you could find books that fill you with joy. If you don't have time to sit down with a book, you could listen to an audio book while feeding your baby.

Some of my mother friends who enjoyed craft would often meet up and have a craft afternoon. For me, I was passionate about nature, green and healthy-living, so I sought out a playgroup at a local community garden. I was also passionate about empowerment, so I organised fundraisers and created affirmations for new mothers during the hours Juan was asleep.

When you come up with some themes, you might like to spend a few nights or a weekend during your pregnancy preparing a scrapbook, picture montage or Pinterest page that honours what you see as your authentic self. When there is literally not a spare second in your chaotic day with your baby, you can leaf through your scrapbook or gaze on images you have collected to remind you of who you are and what you will fully be again in the future.

You don't know yet what life will be like with a baby, so don't set unrealistic expectations. Just become clear about what motivates you outside your professional role, so you can start looking for activities you can do with your baby and partner that fire up those interests.

However, I don't want to discount the role your profession has on you and who you are. During your maternity leave you may wish to maintain a connection with your job, colleagues and industry. Regular lunch dates, visits to the office and even attending networking events (if you're up for it) can keep you in touch with your profession for if and when you're ready to go back to work.

Should I go back to work or stay home?

Deciding whether to return to work, and when, can be a difficult decision. Many women, myself included, believe they will be itching to return to work as soon as possible. However, when our baby arrives our feelings may change.

There is no right or wrong answer about whether you should return to work. For many women, the decision may be financially-driven and you need to work in order to meet financial commitments. Or maybe the availability of childcare options or your level of comfort to leave your baby in the care of others will influence your decision.

Many women return to work as they want to pursue their career or for personal fulfilment. Others who may have previously been career driven may now find fulfilment with full-time mothering. Or perhaps you will find that you have uncovered a new passion or love and want to pursue that. Or you may fit somewhere along that spectrum, and want to balance different elements of the above.

If you decide to return to work, the transition is typically emotional and stressful. You may feel a range of emotions, such as guilt, sadness, excitement and relief. It takes time to adjust, so be gentle on yourself through the process.

While this book doesn't specifically deal with the emotional journey of balancing work and motherhood, many of the connection strategies and exercises included in this book can be used to help in your decision making and transition back to work. In particular, you may wish to use the activities in this *Connect with you* section, which will help you work through the emotional side of the transition. The healing and nurturing activities in *Connect with nature and Maintaining Connections* will also be valuable during this time.

GET CLEAR

'You live out the confusions until they become clear.' – Anais Nin

We're all unique and each of us will have different reasons and combinations of reasons why we decided to become parents. I'm sure there are some of you reading this who have always had clarity about motherhood—you have known your whole life that you wanted to be a mother and you've just been waiting for the right moment. Or maybe your road has been long and arduous, filled with heartache.

For many of us, the reason why we're stepping into motherhood may not be clear. If that's the case, it's important to uncover, clarify and acknowledge the reasons behind your decision to have a baby. You may find that your motivations are creating dangerous expectations about your motherhood journey, and if this is the case it's a good idea to do some emotional healing work before baby arrives.

If you're unsure of your reasons for becoming a mother, the following exercise may help.

\\\\\\\\\\\\\\\\\\\\\\\\\\\\ EXERCISE ////////////////////////

1) Find that special time or place where you do your best thinking. It might be going for a walk, taking a shower or driving your car. While you're in your special place, reflect on the different reasons that led you and your partner to have a baby. It may be straightforward, you may only have one or two reasons. Perhaps you have a lot of different reasons. Be gentle with yourself and have no judgements. This is an exercise in self-discovery and there are no right or wrong responses.

   • Perhaps having a baby is something you think you ought to do. Maybe you're at the stage in life where it's the logical next step. Maybe your friends are transitioning to motherhood and you want to follow suit.
   • Maybe motherhood is an escape. Maybe you've worked so hard that you think having a baby will give you a break, a chance to relax.
   • Perhaps your life has lost some direction or you've gone down a path you no longer like and believe that having a baby might shake things up.
   • Maybe you weren't even expecting to become pregnant; it may have just happened.

2) In your journal, list down all the reasons you can think of.
   For example, for me, if I'm to be truthful, I wasn't sure I wanted to have children, although I was aware that my husband really wanted them and was ready. We were both getting a bit bored with our current routine and felt our lives were self-

focused and indulgent. I was aware that I was creeping into my mid-thirties and should think about starting a family. I also had felt I was a bit off track with where I wanted to be in life, and thought that having a baby might create some chaos that would ultimately allow clarity. It was a combination of all these points that provided the catalyst to try for a baby.

3) Once you have your list, go through and acknowledge your reasons. If you want to deep-dive and explore any of them further, try asking the question 'Why?' Keep asking 'Why?' until you uncover your true motivations. Drilling down to uncover your motivation can help you address any potential disconnection.

4) As you uncover and acknowledge your reasons, think about whether they will support you on this journey or if you need to work through them.

For example, if you find that you want to have a child to relax and take a break from your hectic life, then it's important to understand that up-front. Having a baby usually makes life more hectic and busy, which, if unchecked, may lead to anxiety, stress and disconnection.

5) Finally, think about and list down any action you can take to address areas of disconnection that you have identified.

For example, using the example listed above, maybe you need to explore what makes your life hectic and busy in the first place—are there any patterns? For example, do you say 'yes' to everything and everyone? Can you see yourself taking those patterns into motherhood? To help clear some space in your life and slow down, maybe you need to identify and change some of your patterns. Maybe you can find some support systems to help you when baby comes. It might be worth negotiating an alternative work arrangement for when you're ready to return from maternity leave.

Note, the solutions may not be clear now, but as you go further through the Connection Compass and your pregnancy, you may gain a clearer understanding of what support is required.

\\ ///////////////////////////////////////

If going through the exercise brings up any hurt or pain, I recommend you seek professional help, and now is the time to start that process. For example, you could ask your GP for a referral to a counsellor or use an online directory. Alternatively, you could find an energy healer who can help release any blockages or trauma. Examples of energy healers include emotional release therapists, reiki masters and acupuncturists.

LET GO

Now that you've started to discover the real you and get clear about why you're having a baby, I'm going to contradict myself by asking you to do some letting go. But stick with me; everything will become clear.

Having the ability to let go has tremendous power. It allows us to make room for something new and amazing. To understand how this works you first need to know that everything is made up of energy, including us. Quantum physics has recently discovered this, but the ancients also knew it. Ancient healing practices, such as Chinese qigong, concentrate on the flow of energy and how it affects our lives.

When we hold onto things we don't need—like fears, false beliefs, unresolved issues, unnecessary material possessions—we are holding on to stagnant energy. This blocks our ability to let healthy, life-giving energy enter and flow in our lives.

This isn't great at the best of times, but it can be a real problem when we're transitioning as new parents—a time of constant change, of new beginnings, of uncertainty. This is a time when we need our energy to flow and help us face the changes that unfold.

Now let's go through some of the ways you can let go so that you're open and can allow energy to flow.

Letting go of expectations

'We must be willing to let go of the life we have planned, so as to have the life that is waiting for us.' –Joseph Campbell

We all have expectations. We hold them for events, people, situations, our lives.

Becoming a mother is no different. Over the course of our pregnancy we create all manner of expectations—about how our pregnancy should go, what birth will be like, what our baby will be like, how our partner will be as a father, how we will be as a mother, the activities we'll do when bub arrives.

A lot of our expectation setting is caused by our excitement about becoming a mother and our daydreams about the future. This daydreaming and excitement is a great thing; it starts our bonding process. However, when we form attachments to the daydreams of what *may* be, there is the danger that they will turn into expectations for what *should* be.

This is dangerous because when our reality doesn't live up to our expectations, we feel disappointment. We judge ourselves harshly for it. We may even feel like we have failed.

But we haven't. Our expectations weren't reality; they were merely our beliefs about something we could not have possibly understood until we were there, wearing those shoes.

Babies and everything related to them are unpredictable. Childbirth may be smooth or there may be twists and turns. Some newborns crawl to their mother's breast and latch on first try; others may take several weeks or even months to settle into breastfeeding, if they ever do. Some babies may be dream babies; others may be challenging. Yesterday they may have slept in the car on the way to the shops; today they might scream the whole way. This morning they were happy to lie in the bouncer; this afternoon they only want to be carried.

Holding onto expectations almost always causes disappointment and a feeling that you've lost control. If at all possible, try your best to walk into motherhood with an open mind. If you have beliefs and feelings about what motherhood or your baby or your partner may be like after your transition, leave them at the door. These won't serve you.

Walk into motherhood with this mantra:

'It will be what it will be and I'll meet it from a place of love.'

Letting go of expectations and walking into every situation from a place of openness and allowing flow will be of immeasurable value to your motherhood experience. It's a tool that allows you to be in the driver's seat when it comes to dealing with change, as it allows you to be open to possibilities. It will make you powerful and present to enjoy the moment for what it is and not be fixated on a particular outcome.

I can personally vouch for the fact that fixed expectations can be dangerous. In the fifth month of my pregnancy my husband and I attended a birthing course which opened our eyes to a new way of birthing—a birth that was full of trust and calm. But during my daily preparation of listening to birth affirmations, I consciously shut my mind to the affirmation: 'I calmly accept whatever turn my birthing may take', thinking that the affirmation wasn't going to apply to me. I was headstrong, stubborn even. I was going to have a four-hour natural birth, and there was no way I was going to have a C-section.

Guess what happened? During birth things did not go according to plan, and after fifty-four hours of labour we experienced a twist that led us from midwifery care to obstetrician care. The affirmation that became our mantra from then on was: 'I calmly accept whatever turn my birthing may take', and that turn was ultimately a C-section delivery. Although I'm now at peace with my son's birth, for a long time I felt a sense of disappointment and failure, which could have been avoided if I had not been so headstrong in my expectations of a natural birth.

To many of you, especially those who are action and result oriented (i.e., highly engaged in masculine energy), letting go can be scary. But I'm here to guide you through this experience, and to help you release your expectations.

⧵⧵⧵⧵⧵⧵⧵⧵⧵⧵⧵⧵⧵⧵⧵⧵⧵⧵ EXERCISE ⫻⫻⫻⫻⫻⫻⫻⫻⫻⫻⫻⫻⫻⫻

1) In your journal, draw up two columns. In the first column, write down any expectations or beliefs you're carrying with you. You can use the following questions to prompt some answers:

   - What do you think your pregnancy should be like?
   - What expectations do you have for the birth of your baby?
   - How easy will your baby be to raise?
   - What do you think a typical day will be like when your baby arrives?
   - How do you think your partner will be as a parent?
   - What expectations do you have of your family or your in-laws? Of your friends? Of strangers, even?
   - When will you want to go back to your job?

   Be as truthful as you can.

2) In the second column, for each expectation, think back to the circumstances that led you to form this particular belief. Notice how these circumstances may be giving you false expectations.

   Are they your perceptions of someone else's reality? Are they clouded by fear? Here are some examples:

EXPECTATION	CIRCUMSTANCE
My pregnancy will be easy and a magical time.	Observed the joy and glow of colleagues and friends. (Perception of someone else's reality.)
Motherhood will be the ultimate fulfilment.	Information found in parenting magazines, blogs, conversations with others. (Perception of someone else's reality.)
I will get back to my pre-baby body in a month.	Celebrity magazines and blogs. (Perception of someone else's reality.)
Having a baby will improve my relationship.	Conversations with and observations of friends and family. (Perception of someone else's reality.)
I won't be able to cope with the pain of childbirth.	Stories from friends and colleagues, observations from watching TV and movies and reading books—it seems so painful. (Fear)
The early days of motherhood will be a nightmare. I won't get any sleep and I won't be able to function.	Information read in parenting magazines and blogs. (Fear)

I will have a natural, drug-free birth in four hours.	Friend's experience. (Perception of someone else's reality.)
I will instinctively know how to feed, care for and comfort my baby.	Information read in various media and observation of friends. (Perception of someone else's reality or societal expectations.)
As a mother, I should put my baby's needs first and suck it up if I have any problems.	Information read in various media and observation of other mothers. (Perception of someone else's reality or societal expectations.)
I will be itching to get back to work.	Friend's experience. (Perception of someone else's reality.)

3) By now, hopefully, your expectations are less potent, however, you can further loosen them by saying each of those you've listed out loud and followed by the words:

'It will be what it will be and I'll meet it from a place of love.'

If you do find yourself feeling disappointment about unmet expectations, use gratitude as a healer. Turn your energy to recognising all the things that are positive about the situation or circumstance.

For example, although my son's birth didn't play out as expected, gratitude has helped me to completely accept it. How could I possibly have known that by *not* experiencing the four-hour birth I willed for myself, my life would become so much richer and my passions would be unleashed? I understand now that I had prepared for birth from the masculine, from my mind. Without having the birth that I had, I would not have understood about the power of feminine energy and the importance of being centred in both energies. What a blessing my son's birth turned out to be.

It also helps to communicate your expectations. If the expectation is about the behaviour of a partner or a friend or loved one, it may help to let the other person know your expectation. That way they can either fulfil whatever it is you're hoping to get from them, or work through the issue with you, which will release any pressure from unmet expectations.

Letting go of fear

Fear, by definition, is the intense focusing of our thoughts on something we don't want to happen. I surveyed a number of expectant and new mothers and asked them what they secretly feared. Here are some of their answers:

- 'What if I lose my baby?'
- 'I'm terrified of giving birth.'
- 'I don't know if I can cope with so much pain.'
- 'What if something is wrong with my baby?'
- 'I'm afraid I won't be able to cope when I'm a mother.'
- 'I'm afraid I'm going to do something wrong that will hurt my baby.'
- 'Can we have a baby and survive on one income?'
- 'What will happen to my relationship with my partner? What if we grow apart?'
- 'I'm afraid I won't have a job to come back to from maternity leave.'
- 'I fear the world is getting worse and bringing up children will become more and more difficult.'

- 'I'm afraid of becoming a different person.'
- 'I'm afraid of transferring my fears onto my baby.'
- 'I'm afraid my baby will cry and scream in public and embarrass me.'

From the list above you can tell that facing fears is one of the biggest challenges of motherhood. But it's really important to identify and alchemise the fears that you hold for your pregnancy, birth and early motherhood. Fear will hold you back. It holds us all back. It stops us from being the person, the mother, the role model, the partner, the woman that we want to be. Fear makes us defensive, and prevents us from being true to ourselves. We must learn how to release fear if we want to connect to who we really are. If we don't, we're in danger of becoming something we are not.

As well-known psychologist Dr Phil McGraw often says, 'What you fear, you create.' Our fears become a self-fulfilling prophecy. We have the birth we were afraid of having. Our baby cries in public and embarrasses us. We feel like we're doing it all wrong. We don't have a job to come back to after maternity leave.

So what do we do about fear?

First, you need to understand that you don't have to be afraid of fear. In fact, fear is your friend. There's even a belief that when fears shows up, it's a sign that you're on the right path.

Next, you should understand what the antidote to fear is. We often think the opposite of fear is courage. It's not. The opposite of fear is trust.

To me, learning this provided immense comfort. Trust is something we can have control over and it's a state we can easily create in a matter of minutes if we're able to catch ourselves in a state of fear or worry.

It's helpful to think about times in your life when you have felt fear but have overcome it. If you've overcome fear before, trust that you will be able to overcome and face the fears that arise during your pregnancy, childbirth and early motherhood.

////////////////////////// **EXERCISE** //////////////////////////

1) Find an example of when you have faced your fear.
   - Think back to a time or situation when you felt afraid but chose to face your fear. (For example, I felt fear when I had to abseil off a bridge.)
   - Try to remember how you felt at the time. (My heart raced, I felt panicked, my legs went wobbly, but I was comfortable with the quality of the equipment and my friend's long experience in the sport.)
   - What was the turning point when your fear started to subside? (When I was halfway between the bridge and the ground and I realised I was safe and was actually enjoying myself.)
   - How did you feel afterwards? (I felt proud and elated, like I wanted to do it again.)

Now you have a tangible example to demonstrate that you have the internal resilience and fortitude to face your fears. Knowing that you can overcome your fears, it's now time to identify and release them.

2) Identify your fears.
   - Find a quiet place and write out the things you're worried about or hold secret fears about. Spend some time acknowledging your fear and observe the effect that fear has on your body. Do you tense up? Do you feel something in your stomach? How does fear feel to you?
   - Have a think about whether you have control over each fear you have listed down. For those fears you have some control over, think back to the time you overcame a fear in the past and have trust that you can do it again now and in the future.

3) It's now time to alchemise your fears through a breathing exercise. This is particularly useful for those fears listed that you don't have any control over.

- Close your eyes and breathe in the word 'TRUST or 'I have trust'—whichever feels better for you. Exhale normally.
- After a few breaths, when you exhale, let go of one of the fears on your list.
- Breathe in trust; exhale your fear. Repeat until you no longer feel the sensation of fear.
- Move on to your next fear and repeat this process.

\\ ////////////////////////////////////

In the future, whenever a fear pops up and you feel the fear sensation, you can use the above exercise to alchemise the fear.

Just a final word on fear and having trust. If you feel fear that is outside of your control, then trust comes from knowing that no matter what the outcome is, you will be able to get through it. That you will have the support you need and the inner resilience to come out the other side.

When you let go of expectations and fears, you will find that you will more deeply connect with your true self. Expectations and fears are energy in the form of thoughts and emotions that cloud your true self; they are not who you really are.

SET INTENTIONS

'Energy flows where intention goes.' –James Redfield

Imagine if you started a journey with no directions and only a vague idea of where you wanted to go. You would probably wander around aimlessly. You'd waste time; you'd become frustrated. It would also take you a lot longer to reach your destination. Just because I've asked you to do some letting go, doesn't mean that I want you to enter your motherhood journey without any kind of plan. And now that you've cleared the air, it's a good time to think about setting some guiding principles.

I'm sure you're more than familiar with goal-setting, which is how most people address this problem. But setting goals in motherhood can be dangerous for your emotional and mental wellbeing because it depends on your being in control, and when you become a parent you'll find out that many things are outside your control. For example, setting a goal such as 'I will have a drug-free labour' or 'I will drop back to my pre-baby weight in six weeks' can set you up to feel failure and disillusionment if circumstances prevent you from meeting your goal.

As professional women, it's important during pregnancy and motherhood to step outside the goal-setting mentality we've grown so accustomed to and adapt an intention-setting mentality instead. Intention-setting is a little different from goal-setting. Goals are concerned with a fixed outcome, which we either achieve or don't. An intention is a guiding principle that you have with you at all times and can invoke at any moment.

Deepak Chopra describes intentions as 'directed impulses of consciousness that contain the seed of that which you aim to create.'[4] Intentions still provide guidance and direction, but they aren't defined by the outcome; instead they are dynamic and adaptive.

Here are some examples of how a defined goal can become a more realistic guiding principle or intention:

- 'I will have a healthy and straightforward pregnancy' could be replaced with 'I allow my body to go through the miraculous changes involved in growing a healthy baby.'
- 'I will have a drug-free labour' could be replaced with 'I am confident in my ability to calmly and safely birth my baby.'

- 'I will drop back to my pre-baby weight in six weeks' could be replaced with 'I will give my body the best chance possible to safely recover after the amazing changes in pregnancy and birth.'
- 'I will have the same relationship with my partner as I do now' could be replaced with 'My relationship with my partner evolves as we both find our feet as parents.'

Although they may sound wishy-washy, especially if you're used to setting specific and measurable goals, setting intentions will help you gain clarity for your motherhood journey while allowing you to have flexibility. You will evolve as your pregnancy progresses as well as when your baby arrives, and the beauty about intentions is that you can change and evolve them also as you grow.

EXERCISE

1) Follow the meditation provided on page 149 so you can step into your intention setting from a state of restful awareness and let go of any negative chatter.

2) When you come out of meditation, set your intentions. You can use the following questions as prompts:
   - What kind of pregnancy do I want?
   - What kind of labour and birth do I want?
   - Who do I want to be as a mother?
   - What kind of relationship do I want with my child?
   - What kind of relationship do I want with my partner?
   - How do I want to balance motherhood and career aspirations?

   Here are a few tips for setting intentions:
   - Make them meaningful to you.

- Use the present tense of the end result (i.e. I am, rather than I will).
- Make them expansive; think big.
- Ensure they're achievable and believable to you.
- Use positive language.
- Use empowering words.
- Make them clear and concise.

3) Write your intentions in your journal and on Post-it notes to stick where you will see them every day, such as the bathroom mirror. You may even wish to record them on your smartphone so you can play them back to yourself.

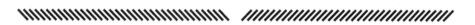

While it's important to regularly remind yourself of your intentions, also try to detach from them. Don't force an outcome. Allow what needs to be to be.

BE AWARE OF YOUR EMOTIONS

The transition into motherhood is an emotionally charged time as creating new life encourages an opening of your heart. A great deal of unexpected emotions may surface for you. You may experience mood swings, feeling elated and excited one minute and worried and fearful the next. It's wonderful to allow and acknowledge this opening of your heart and be gentle and accepting of yourself and your changing feelings.

This can be particularly difficult for those of us working in professions where we are used to operating from our head, not our heart. For a great majority of us, we have learnt to suppress and sometimes avoid emotions in order to succeed in our work, and instead function through rationality and reason. But in order to fully connect with yourself, try to get in touch with your emotions and become comfortable experiencing strong emotions and their fluctuations.

This is important for both yourself and your baby. It's important for you because it allows you to be present and to honour and listen to your emotions, which in turn improves both your mental and physical well-being. Psychologist Jonathan Adler and Hal E. Hershfield, Professor of marketing at New York University, undertook research on the link between mixed emotional experiences and psychological welfare. They concluded that: 'Taking the good and bad together may detoxify the bad experiences, allowing you to make meaning out of them in a way that supports psychological well-being.'[5] It might sound counter-intuitive, but it's crucially important to understand that when you accept a negative emotion, it tends to lose its destructive power.

Emotions are also intrinsically linked with physical health. By feeling and accepting the emotional swings that come with the transition to motherhood—kindly and without judgement—you can reduce stress and improve your immune system, which helps your general wellbeing.

Getting in touch with your emotions is important for your baby because the state of your mind is mirrored in your baby's developing brain and nervous system. While emotions don't cross the placenta, the hormones associated with them do, and this includes cortisol, the hormone released during stress.[6]

When a mother is calm and relaxed, so is her baby. Similarly, babies pick up on their mothers' feelings of being angry, anxious, afraid or upset. It's even been shown that a baby's heart rate can double in response to any fright and anxiety that her mother feels.[7] The worry, stress and anxiety that mothers experience during pregnancy has been shown to increase the chances of giving birth to babies who are irritable and experience gastrointestinal troubles and, in some studies, lower cognitive development scores.[8]

It's important to be mindful of how you absorb and cope with stress. Short-term emotional upsets and ordinary day-to-day stress aren't likely to cause any long-term problems for your baby, but it's another story for major emotional disturbances and excessive worry and stress. The key to preventing stress from getting out of hand is to be mindful and aware of your state of mind and how you feel. You don't even need to *understand* what is happening to your emotions. Just having an *awareness* will help.

I read about this when I was pregnant and the knowledge was highly influential on my pregnancy. I became an emotional ninja— when an external drama, stressful situation or something overtly negative came within a five-metre radius, I observed it and then kicked it away. I felt it but didn't entertain it. This didn't stop the swing of emotions that came up as a result of my heart opening, but through mindfulness and awareness of the emotion I was able to cope with it in a psychologically and physically healthy way.

I knew that my emotions and energy were inextricably linked to my son and it was my job as his mother to protect and nurture him and give him the best start in life that I possibly could.

The power of acceptance

During this tender and precious time of opening, it's often the acknowledgement and acceptance of your emotions that can provide great healing and comfort.

One of my favourite mantras, which I adopted from Esther Hicks and use whenever I feel out of whack, is:

'I am where I am and it's okay.'

In other words, acknowledge how you feel and accept it. It's okay to feel the way you feel. This gives you the freedom to move on to a better-feeling place—or if you're already in a great place, you can stay where you are with joy.

\\\\\\\\\\\\\\\\\\\\\\\\\ EXERCISE ////////////////////////

1) Over the next five days, be mindful of your thoughts, your emotions and the words you use. Can you spot any trends? Are your thoughts/words/emotions mainly negative or positive? That is, do they make you feel worse or do they make you feel better? Are they a combination of the two?

2) At the end of the five days:

If you're feeling good and everything seems to be going well, reflect on what happened that made you feel good. Was it external influences? Internal influences? If you haven't already, see if you can build those influences into your daily routine.

If you observe a pattern of feeling anxious, stressed, agitated, worried or overly emotional at the end of the five days, there are likely some blockages or fears that you need to address.

Continue monitoring your emotions and thoughts, remaining aware and alert to what is going on within and around you.

\\\\\\\\\\\\\\\\\\\\\\\\\\\\\\\\\ ////////////////////////////////

As you continue to read this book you will find a number of activities that can help you reduce your stress levels and find a place of centredness and calm. We started this process when we looked at letting go of fears and expectations. *Connect with nature* shows the healing benefits of spending time in nature. The final section of this book, *Maintaining connections,* contains a menu of simple activities guaranteed to make you feel better.

If you find there are still issues that you think need additional attention, such as persistent anxiety or some deep-rooted fears, you may wish to consult your care provider, an energy healer or a counsellor.

Take the TV and news detox challenge

There are many factors that influence your emotional health and a big one is watching and buying into 'the news'. Psychologists have known about this for a long time, and studies undertaken by Dr Graham Davey, PhD, in 1997 demonstrated that people who watched negative news bulletins reported being significantly more anxious and sadder than those who watched neutral or positive news bulletins. Not only that, they were also more likely to catastrophise, and personal worries and concerns that weren't even related to the content of the programme they watched were exacerbated.[9]

Go on a bad-news detox for a week. Turn off the TV and stop watching and reading the news. See how that makes you feel. Trust me, your baby will thank you for it when there are no hormones associated with negative emotions crossing the placenta.

I can hazard a guess that you're protesting—you need to know what's going on in the world. I used to be a major TV and news junkie, but about eight years ago I went cold turkey on both TV and news. I haven't missed out on the news I need to know as it always filters through to me. The benefits are tremendous; I no longer take on the negativity and anger that floods the media with stories that actually have no bearing on my life or my family.

Try it for a week and see what differences it makes to your emotional state.

Coping with loss

Unfortunately miscarriage and stillbirth is a reality that many of us face in our pregnancies. The loss of our baby is devastating. Not only do we lose our precious baby, but also the hopes and dreams for that baby.

The loss of a baby brings up a host of emotions, which may vary from day to day. According to Terry Diamond[10], a perinatal bereavement counsellor, it can be common to have good days and then bad days and this is part of the healing process.

If you're faced with loss, here are some ideas that can be helpful:

- Share your experience with people you love and trust, or a health professional. Talking about what happened can help you process your experience.
- Practice self care. This may include taking time off to work to heal, getting lots of sleep (if possible), eating well and taking time for gentle exercise. Meditation and journaling may also help. Do things that are gentle and kind to yourself and your heart.
- Consider taking a short break. Getting away for a few days may help you heal. When I experienced a miscarriage, my husband and I spent a couple of days away in nature for a change of scenery to share our emotions and be away from reminders of our loss.
- If it feels right, you may wish to do something special to mark the miscarriage. For example, a ceremony or blessing for your baby.

HONOUR YOUR BODY

The next step in connecting with yourself involves developing a greater awareness of your body and understanding the important role it's about to play in your life. When you conceive, gestate and give birth to a child, your body goes through amazing and dramatic changes. It's important to remember, however, that your body is well equipped for this experience and, in fact, was designed for it. Yet there are a number of things you can do to give your body (and mind) a helping hand.

Keeping active

Exercise is really important for the journey into motherhood. While exercise has many physical benefits, it also has emotional benefits. Exercise makes you feel better by releasing chemicals known as endorphins that raise your mood. It's also an important way of connecting with yourself. As you get out of your mind and into your body, you become more balanced and closer to your true self.

It's advisable to discuss your exercise routine with your care provider, but a golden rule is not to try a new sport or take your exercise to another level during pregnancy. Instead, try to maintain your current level of activity. You should also be careful not to exert yourself too much during pregnancy and the first six or so weeks of motherhood. Your body requires some time to heal after giving birth, so low-impact activities such as walking are advisable.

Before having Juan I used to enjoy running, swimming and cycling and would go to the gym every other day. During my pregnancy I jogged for a while and kept up the swimming, but stopped cycling when my baby bump got in the way. Every day I would make sure I had twenty minutes of exercise, whether that was going for a walk before work or during my lunch break, or going to the gym for a low impact workout. I also practised prenatal yoga.

However, when my son arrived I had trouble getting out and doing the amount of exercise I was used to. I had no-one to leave Juan with during the day, and couldn't go to the gym or even take a quick thirty-minute run. Instead I'd take Juan for a walk every day, either in the pram or strapped to my chest in a baby carrier. He loved the movement and being out and about, and would often fall asleep instantly. If he stayed awake he loved looking at the contrast of colours in nature, especially trees.

We also danced. Dancing made me happy, and allowed me to exercise in the privacy of my home while bonding with my son and raising both his mood and mine.

There are structured exercise classes that incorporate prenatal and postnatal support, bonding and connection as well as fitness regimes. These include yoga classes, fitness classes and kangatraining (where you exercise with bub in a carrier). These activities allow you to exercise in a manner that supports your pre- and post-natal body, bond with your baby, and meet other mums. Some gyms and pools also offer a crèche service where your baby can be looked after while you get some exercise. Another idea is to organise informal exercise groups with some of your mother friends and take it in turns to look after the children.

Get your exercise on

If you set a realistic intention you're more likely to achieve it. So instead of making a vague promise to keep fit during your transition to motherhood, try to plan how to get twenty minutes of exercise at least three times a week. You may have to be inventive, but remember that exercise does not have to be sport-based. See what activities you can do at or around the home that can become a normal part of your routine. For example, walking up to the local shops to get some bread, milk and nappies. Incidental exercise and simply being physically active are just as crucial as a formal exercise routine.

Training for labour

It's common as professionals to 'live in our heads'. Therefore being in touch with and trusting our bodies is something we need to train for. Like training for a once-in-a-lifetime trek in the Himalaya or running a marathon, we also need to train for childbirth. Our training involves learning how to relax and be in our bodies. It's really a lot easier (and some may argue more enjoyable) than training for a marathon or a big trek.

The reason why a lot of women fear birth is because of the pain. However, experience and science have proven it's a cycle, and a cycle can be broken. If you have fear, your body will cramp up and cause pain when you have a contraction. When the next contraction hits, you'll fear the coming pain, causing your body to cramp up more and make you feel even more pain. And then the next time you have a contraction, you feel even more fear of the coming pain and your body cramps up even more and so on and so on. This cycle of pain is termed the Fear-Tension-Pain cycle.

When you feel fear, your body goes into fight or flight mode. Blood and oxygen rush from non-essential organs to key organs. Unfortunately, your uterus is not essential for your survival, which is fine if you're being chased by a tiger, but not very good if you're giving birth.

As explained in Marie Mongan's book, *HypnoBirthing: the Mongan Method*,[11] the uterus has three layers of muscles. The outer layer has muscles that run vertically and are aligned with your baby. The inner layer has horizontal circular layers that surround your baby. The inner layers are found mostly at the lower part of the uterus, just above the cervix.

To release your baby, the cervix needs to dilate, or open. When this happens, the outer layer of uterine muscles draws the circular layers up to allow the cervix to soften and thin. This movement is what is known as contractions, but a less confronting way of describing it is surges.

If you feel fear or tension when the surges happen, the blood rushes away from your uterus and this process becomes intensely painful. The normal practice is to offer drugs and pain relief to help dull the senses. However, there is a kinder and gentler way, which is to create a calm environment for childbirth, relax, move and breathe through your surges. Use your voice to sound out the waves with your breath if you'd like to. The sensations are still intense but manageable.

It works. Recent research by Western Sydney University and the National Institute of Complementary Medicine studied women who followed the SheBirths program, using holistic, relaxing techniques, such as relaxation, yoga, visualisation, massage and acupressure. Results showed that during labour, those women had a 65% reduction in epidural rates and a 44% reduction in caesarean sections as compared to the control group[12].

Relaxation, touch (when desired) and other holistic birth techniques help the natural stimulation of birth hormones. Oxytocin causes the uterus to contract and helps dilate and thin the cervix to move baby down the birthing path. Endorphins are our natural pain-killers and during birth will bring you into an altered state. As labour progresses naturally, more oxytocin is released, causing further surges which, in turn, increase the production of endorphins. The more intense the surges and resulting sensations, the more the endorphin levels rise in response.[13]

This was reflected in my own birth experience, where I let go of fear and embraced holistic birthing techniques. I listened to calm music and visualisations, enjoyed soft massage, breathed and danced my way through sixty-two hours of surges. Yet I also know what happens when you let the fear in. There were about ten minutes during my labour when I lost my cool. During those minutes I felt excruciating pain. It wasn't fun. But I did get my cool back.

While my son's birth was not without twists and turns, it was a beautiful experience. During the lead up to birth I had equipped myself with tools to remain calm and had practised diligently daily, just as I had once exercised and run daily in preparation for a half-marathon.

The following are approaches that may help you train for labour.

Hypnobirthing

Hypnobirthing uses a breathing technique to help you breathe through the surges or contractions of labour. It's great to practice this daily so you know how to access the breath when you need it during labour.

Slowly inhale and count quickly for as long as you can (up to the count of sixteen or twenty if possible) and exhale slowly to the same count. If your surge hasn't passed, just repeat this breath until it has.[14] This is a wonderfully effective breathing technique and has worked for countless thousands of women each year.

We used the relaxation techniques of hypnobirthing, such as soft massage, breathing exercises, hypnosis exercises, affirmations and visualisations, to prepare for Juan's birth because they resonated with us. We especially liked that hypnobirthing provided techniques that allowed Leland to be an active participant in the labour process.

Active birth

Active birth is a method that involves mothers learning to follow their instinctive movements during labour and birth. It encourages you to be active in your labour and choose positions freely, for example, walking around, remaining upright, squatting or whatever other position feels right at the time. This can be especially important for when baby is in posterior and breech positions, because movement can help turn the baby into a better position and, therefore, reduce the risk of medical intervention. Active birth makes the most of gravity and provides opportunities to involve both parents in the labour and birthing process. Its benefits include a less painful labour and better oxygen flow to the baby.[15]

Prenatal yoga

Prenatal yoga explores movement, physical postures, breathing, sound, relaxation and visualisation as a way to meet the needs of pregnant women. It offers an opportunity to cultivate a closer relationship with your body, mind and heart and a special time to bond with your baby.[16]

SheBirths

The SheBirths program[17] is based a philosophy of knowledge, inner strength and outer support. Preparations for birth incorporate elements from prenatal yoga, active birth, hypnosis, acupressure, massage, visualisation, pain management and nutrition.

Each of the above birth preparations can be used separately or in conjunction with each other.

CREATE ENERGY

Almost every pregnant woman and new mother I surveyed said they wanted more time. Pregnant women wanted more time to prepare. New mothers wanted more time in their day to get things done, more time to themselves, and more time to just enjoy being with their baby.

Unfortunately, we cannot create more time. Each of us has twenty-four hours in a day, seven days in a week. But what if I threw it out there that having more time might not actually be the answer to fitting more into our day?

What if managing our energy was actually the answer? Unlike time, we can create more of it. Energy is a renewable resource, and we all have ways in which we can expand and renew our energy. Because we're all made up of energy, finding ways to create more energy also forges a stronger connection with ourselves. And when we increase that connection, in turn, we find even more energy.

In the early days of motherhood our energy levels are typically low. Birthing our babies takes a lot out of us, and in the blur of the first couple of weeks and months we may experience lack of sleep, lack of exercise, inadequate nutrition and fluctuating emotions. It's a good idea to learn how to manage your energy levels *before* having your baby so you can keep them as high as possible during this critical time.

Managing your energy is two-fold: It's crucial that you expend your available energy in the right way, and that you find ways to re-energise.

To make sure you're expending your energy on the right things, it's important that your priorities suit what's right for you. Prioritising your activities and cutting back what's unnecessary can allow you to spend energy (and, implicitly, time) on yourself—whether that means having a nap, getting some exercise, getting out of the house and getting some fresh air or taking a bath. Whatever will make you feel better in yourself.

EXERCISE

1) Be conscious about how you're spending your time and energy. For the next three days, write down all the things you do in a day, and how much time you spend on each activity.

   For example: working, cooking, cleaning, groceries, Facebook/ social media, watching television, spending time with your partner and friends, exercising, etc.

2) From that list, work out which activities are actually necessary and add a lot of value to your day. Work out what activities are sapping your energy or not making you feel good.

3) Cut out the activities that are not necessary. Be brutal.

For example, do you really have to make the bed every day? Does it matter if the roses aren't pruned? Does spending fifteen minutes on Instagram enrich your day?

4) For those non-essential activities, work out what can you do to cut them back (or out completely) or delegate them. Who can come and help you?

For example, can you cook big batches of food once a week and freeze for later? When bub arrives, can you ask friends or family to prepare meals for you? Can you hire a cleaner to come in a few hours a week or can your partner do the cleaning? Or can you both do power bursts of cleaning for ten minutes a day so it doesn't pile up? Can you order your groceries and other shopping online and have them delivered? Can you allocate specific times of the day to connect with social media?

5) Once you've scaled back the activities that sap your energy, what activities can you replace them with? I.e. what activities power you and make you feel good?

For example, instead of watching television, you might want to have a bath, read a book or do some stretches. When bub arrives and is sleeping, instead of doing housework you might want to use that time to do things for yourself. For example, writing a journal, doing a daily project (we did a 365 day photo blog of our son's first year), gardening, etc.

Replenishing your energy can be quite simple and with some practice you can power up quickly. Simple ways of re-energising include:

- Breathing exercises
- Meditation
- Expressing gratitude and appreciation of others

The last section of the book focuses on techniques to help you energise and stay centred and grounded. Find methods that resonate with you and can fit into your schedule, and stick with them. Remember that it's much easier to continue these exercises if you have already set up a ritual during pregnancy.

Power up with good nutrition

Nutrition is important for increasing energy levels. Pregnancy and breastfeeding take a lot out of your body, so try to ensure you're fuelling your body with as much nutritious and healthy food as possible. I found when my son was a newborn I had trouble eating properly during the day. It was fine when my husband was home and could tend to Juan's needs while I prepared our evening meal, but during the day I'd find myself halfway through preparing lunch and then Juan would need feeding and it could be several hours before I could get back to my meal.

Being organised will help here:

- Have fruit and vegetable sticks pre-cut in the fridge so you can grab some healthy snacks when you need them. You can buy these in the supermarket if you don't have time to cut them yourself.
- Pre-cook meals for lunch, or cook extra the night before so you can just reheat the next day.

Get in the habit of stocking fresh, healthy, highly nutritious foods in the fridge so that you can throw together a meal in a few minutes with minimal preparation. Foods that can be eaten as a snack or thrown together as a quick salad include:

- Veggies such as avocadoes, cherry tomatoes and baby spinach leaves.
- Proteins such as yoghurt, cottage cheese, tuna or boiled eggs.
- Starch and carbohydrates such as brown rice cakes and wholemeal wraps.
- Seeds such as chia, pepita and sunflower.
- Nuts such as almond, walnut, cashew and macadamia.

Protein-rich foods and complex carbohydrates provide lasting energy, so get in the habit of stocking those in your fridge and cupboards if you don't already. Try to eat wholefoods, and buy organic where possible. It's tempting to keep processed and high-sugar foods in your pantry as an easy option, but they only provide short-term energy spikes followed by an energy crash.

Eating nutritious food in the morning is especially important as it sets up your energy levels for the day. Try to start your day with meals that you can throw together in a matter of minutes, such as oats, sugar-free yoghurt, berries, shredded coconut, banana, seeds and nuts (being mindful of any allergies your bub may have).

Get moving for more energy

I talked about keeping active earlier and want to reiterate that exercise is important for replenishing your energy. Doing some stretches or prana (energy) cleansing movements (see page 152) can help boost your energy in a matter of minutes. The prana cleansing movements are especially good as the symmetrical and fluid movements help balance and centre both the masculine and feminine energies, which can help you remain grounded during this chaotic time. The exercise I have listed in the back of the book only requires a few minutes.

De-clutter

De-cluttering your home is another way of boosting your energy levels. As they're predominantly stagnant in nature, the physical and material possessions we own can actually drain our energy.

It's unsurprising, then, that many women feel an urge to clean and purge the house during the final weeks of pregnancy in an expression of their 'nesting instinct'.

I didn't really understand about possessions holding stagnant energy until my son was about five or six months old. I realised that soon he would start moving about independently and there was a real danger that he might pull furniture down on himself.

When I assessed our house and furniture, I realised the only major risk was my prized bookshelf, which held carefully chosen books collected over time and on my travels, but which couldn't be fixed to the wall.

I made a decision. The bookshelf had to go and so did the books. Before I could change my mind, I piled the books into boxes and we drove across the city and donated them to a community bookstore that gave the proceeds of sales to charity.

I kept a handful of books that I felt still had a purpose—ones that weren't holding stagnant energy—but everything else was given away. It felt amazing. I had been holding on to years and years' worth of books, taking them with me from city to city, sometimes even country to country, without realising I was holding on to stagnant energy. When I gave them away, we experienced a tangible shift in energy, and more seemed to flow into our home. I never once regretted giving away my books or, to be honest, even missed them.

When letting go of the clutter in your house, ask yourself these questions:

- Is there anything you've been intending to do but have been putting off?

- Is there a section of your home that is full of clutter? Maybe it's your kitchen drawers or bathroom cabinets.
- Are you holding on to old mementos that you no longer need?
- What possessions in your home can you live without?

De-clutter time

Find a corner of your house that could do with some spring cleaning. Be brutal. Be ruthless. Ask yourself if you really need to keep an item or whether it's holding stagnant energy. If the item is sentimental, consider taking a photo before disposing of it. I find it can be easier to let go of items when you have your partner, a family member or a friend helping you. They probably don't have the same attachments as you do and will be able to help you determine what's clutter and what's worth keeping.

De-cluttering will help you increase your energy levels, but it's also the last and most important step in connecting with yourself. When you remove clutter, you pare yourself back and can more clearly see your true self. With the mess cleared away, there is nowhere to hide, but you also realise that you're defined not by material possessions, but by what is in your heart and soul.

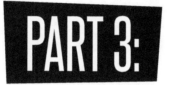

PART 3:

CONNECT WITH YOUR BABY

Attachment to a baby is a long-term process, not a single, magical moment.

T. BERRY BAZELTON

The connection between you and your baby starts now and lasts a lifetime. The more you go inwards and connect with your baby during pregnancy, the better start you give her in life. It will also help prepare you as you step into your role as mother—as you engage with your nurturing and mothering side. Connecting with your baby doesn't just foster a relationship with your baby; it also allows you to further connect with yourself.

Feel free to bookmark this section and give it to your partner to read. The great majority of these ideas can be used by fathers and partners too, helping them to form deep and lifelong bonds with their baby.

BOND FROM THE BEGINNING

The connection that parents form with their babies is known as bonding or forming positive attachment. Bonding is how babies— before and after birth—discover and learn what the world is all about.

Forming connections with your baby, throughout pregnancy and when your baby arrives, is a wonderful investment in your child's emotional development and gives them a great start in life. A secure bond gives your baby the optimal foundation for life, as their sense of well-being, acceptance and esteem as a welcome and loved person are being formed during this time.

During pregnancy, birth and early motherhood, if not interfered with, nature unlocks reciprocal bonded patterns between mother and baby, such as biorhythms, heart frequencies, hormonal balances and sleep patterns. Your baby provides the precise stimulus for you to open and develop new capabilities and you provide the same stimulus for your baby.

However, you can do much to help and enhance this natural process, and this section will go through the different ways you and your partner can connect and bond with your baby to form positive and secure attachment.

Pregnancy

Preparation is key to a calm transition to motherhood, and you can use the months of pregnancy to begin enhancing your natural connection with your baby. The months your baby spends inside your womb are a tremendous opportunity to connect with him or her.

Mothers tend to bond first, as they feel the changes in their body. For many fathers, the connection becomes real when they hear their baby's heart beat and see their child during ultrasounds. Some mothers intuitively feel connected to their baby right from the moment he's conceived. For other parents, the feeling grows as the baby develops and, for many, it becomes especially prominent when they feel the baby kick for the first time. This is further enhanced when they can feel their baby's movement in response to their voice and music.

Dr Thomas Verny, a leading authority on the effect of prenatal and early postnatal environment on personality development, sees the core of human personality forming not during the first three years of life, as commonly believed, but rather in the womb.[18] During pregnancy, your body provides sensory stimulation that is associated with shaping your baby's brain. This stimulation may be through touch or through sound. Dr Verny maintains that new brain cells are being formed constantly and create pathways and circuits for the baby's development. Stimulation develops those pathways and makes them stronger, meaning that when your child is born, they're better prepared for the world.[19]

Research also shows that babies in the womb have the emotional and intuitive capabilities to sense their parents' love. According to Carista Luminare-Rosen, author and founder of *The Centre for Creative*

Parenting in California, prenatal babies can see, hear, feel, remember, taste and think before birth.[20]

Bonding with your child during pregnancy also helps you, your partner and other family members to prepare emotionally for the new addition to the family. Through interacting and playing with the baby in utero, a relationship and trust starts forming and the baby becomes quite real. There is truly nothing more magical than feeling your baby respond to you and having two-way communication through the womb.

Birth and beyond

Your baby's birth is a co-created act—it's a process that you go through together. Unless labour is started through induction or the birth is a pre-planned caesarean section, your baby will usually instigate the process. Labour is also a time when you can increase the bonds between yourself and your baby. You and your partner can talk to your baby during birth, telling him that he's doing a wonderful job and that you're excited to meet him. You can sing to him, welcome him. Listening to calming music during labour will help relax both you and your baby, while invigorating music is appropriate for the more active stage of transition and birth.

Careful preparation for labour will help mitigate the pain and stress involved. This, in turn, helps you connect with baby by allowing hormones to be released that encourage bonding. Feeling calm, safe, nurtured and supported are conditions that encourage the natural production of birth hormones.

Science is now proving what ancient cultures have known for a long time. The manner in which your baby is welcomed into the world during the first hours after birth may have short- and long-term impacts on their development.

Just for a moment, think about this transition from your baby's point of view. For nine months your baby has been safe in a completely controlled, fluid-filled sac. She has never experienced direct light, temperature changes or hunger. Now, all of a sudden, she's out in the world and everything that she has known has changed. It takes a while for a baby to adjust to their new reality and home. You can help her by doing everything you can to quickly develop an intimate connection.

In order to make the transition from the womb to the outside world as calm and peaceful as possible for all parties, there are a number of attachment practices that your whole family can do in the first hours and days. For example, skin-to-skin contact, breastfeeding, talking, singing and cuddling. These are discussed later under *Bond with the five senses*.

It's worth noting that connecting with your baby immediately after birth may not come as easily as you expect. You may or may not feel the profound love that you expect to feel. You may be tired or you may still be coming to terms with your birth experience, or there may be health considerations that cause distress or concern.

Luckily, nature plays a large role in aiding the bonding process. Nature assumes that a mother and child bond will develop by placing a baby close to their mother's body and breast for an extended period of time. Nature intends that intimate contact between a baby and her mother's body will provide pleasurable stimulation and emotional nurturing, as well as the essential nutrients needed to develop a normal brain and nervous system.

As you spend more time with your baby and get to know him, connecting becomes easier. As you understand and become more responsive to your baby's communication, such as his cries and body language, the stronger your connection will become and the easier it will be.

There are many ways to bond with your baby, including feeding your baby, massage, play, movement, reading and singing to your baby, structured classes such as baby sensory, kangatraining and mums and bubs yoga. To make bonding as complete as possible, let's now look at how to use all five of our senses in the bonding process.

BOND WITH THE FIVE SENSES

Some means of bonding with your baby may seem obvious—everybody knows how to cuddle and coo over a baby. But cuddling and cooing are limited ways of using just two of our five senses. As adults, we rely a lot on language to communicate, but while a baby can verbally communicate by crying and gurgling and so forth, she does not have the power of language to help her. So she relies equally on all five senses to be fully nourished, nurtured, supported and protected by her caregivers.

Using the full five senses allows for both an emotional and biological attachment between you and your baby. Setting up these positive attachments has lifetime benefits for your child, as it sets them up for developing trust, confidence, and a sense of place and belonging. The attachment they form as babies will also shape their expectations in later relationships.

So that you can connect with your baby in a more complete way, let's now go through how to use all five of your senses and your baby's senses to help you bond and set up positive attachment, both before and after birth.

TOUCH

Michelangelo once said, 'To touch can be to give life.' Research is suggesting that touch is truly fundamental to human communication, bonding and health.[21] Touch is important for your baby's development as it stimulates growth hormones and relieves stress hormones. It enhances your baby's feeling of being loved and helps contribute to her self-esteem. It also activates the orbitofrontal cortex in your baby's brain, which is linked to feelings of reward and compassion, and the vagus nerve, which is intimately involved with her compassionate response. Touch is soothing; it signals safety and trust and can also trigger the release of oxytocin.[22]

Pregnancy

Touch is the first sense to develop, just days after conception, and is important for your child's whole lifetime. At just seven weeks after conception, your baby responds to your twists and turns with movements of her own. At twelve weeks, she kicks. At sixteen weeks, she begins to suck her thumb. By her sixth month, her kicks, somersaults, twists and turns are very noticeable and powerful.

The urge to stroke your belly and stimulate your child tactilely is innate—communicating with your unborn child through touch is as old as humanity itself. From the time your baby grows enough for you to feel her everyday movements, which is typically between week eighteen and twenty-two, you can start to communicate with her through touch.

The wonderful thing about bonding through touch is that you can have two-way communication. You can send your baby a message and she can give you a response. When that happens, it's the most magical feeling. I often felt like my son and I belonged to a secret club. I would be in meetings at the office and my baby and I were communicating to each other via touch and movement that no-one else knew about or noticed.

You can use touch to communicate with your baby in a number of ways:

- Press down gently on your belly.
- Rub your baby bump in circular movements or from side to side.
- Gently tap and drum your fingers on your stomach.

Then feel how your baby responds to your touch. This may be through kicking her legs, nudging with her elbow, or twisting and turning her body. If she doesn't respond immediately, don't worry, she may just be having a nap. But if at any time you're worried about your baby's movements or if you notice a change in your baby's pattern of movement, call your care provider so you can check on her well-being.

When bub arrives

As well as communicating with your baby using the techniques described earlier, you can work with your baby during birth by moving your body. Active birth and prenatal yoga techniques are great for connecting with your baby during birth and are useful for turning your baby into a more optimal position if needed. Many women, including myself, dance their babies into the world, using intuitive movement. If you turn off your mind chatter and tune into your body, it knows how to move during this sacred dance of birth. You have probably danced with your partner many times to express and reinforce your connection, and it works the same way with your baby, even before he or she is born.

In the hospital

Skin-to-skin contact with your baby immediately after birth helps your baby make the transition to newborn life easier from both a physical and emotional perspective.

Skin-to-skin contact promotes the flow of oxytocin, the 'love hormone', which helps both you and your baby fall in love with each other. This can also reduce the stress your baby may feel after transitioning through labour and birth.

Skin-to-skin contact promotes greater respiratory and glucose stability. Your body actually regulates its temperature based on your baby's temperature and will heat up or cool down depending on what your baby requires. Your skin also contains microbiomes, or beneficial bacteria, which are essential to the health of your baby. When your baby is placed skin-to-skin, they're exposed to healthy bacteria which helps strengthen their immune system.

Being skin-to-skin also encourages breastfeeding, as it allows your baby to follow their instincts and scent to your breast.

The benefits aren't just for babies. Mothers who hold their babies skin-to-skin have increased maternal behaviours, show more confidence in caring for their baby and may breastfeed for longer durations.

This is really important to know as medical protocol can often interfere with skin-to-skin contact. Advise your caregivers that you want skin-to-skin contact immediately after birth so the hospital can modify their procedures to allow this. Other than convenience or a legitimate health concern, there is no need for the hospital to rush the birth of the placenta or pressure you to have the baby weighed and measured. After the crucial first hour or so has passed, you can continue skin-to-skin contact. If you breastfeed, this helps facilitate ongoing skin-to-skin contact.

Skin-to-skin contact is not just for mothers. It also helps fathers form an attachment with their baby in the first few days and weeks. This will be a special time for them to get to know their baby, and while they bond it gives you time to rest and recharge your batteries.

At home

You won't need to be reminded to kiss and cuddle your baby, but you might like to know that kissing and cuddling does more than express your love. After my son Juan was born, I was compelled to kiss him every chance I could get. Some days I felt like I was a kissing machine. He was just so kissable. I figured it was because I was head over heels in love with him. On an unconscious level I supposed that kissing him was forming an emotional attachment for both of us.

That is all quite true, but it turns out nature also had a role to play in protecting his physical health. As Juan was a breastfed baby, kissing him was actually protecting him from the pathogens he was exposed to. My lips were taking in those pathogens, as were my secondary lymphoid organs (such as my tonsils), where memory B cells specific for those pathogens were formed. My breasts used those memory B cells to produce antibodies for those pathogens. When I nursed Juan, he received the antibodies via my breast milk. It's absolutely mind-blowing—who knew an expression of love could do so much. I'm not sure why I was surprised to learn this, as the more I dug, the more I found that nature has a hand in most things when it comes to connecting with your baby.

As well as the natural acts of cuddling, kissing and hugging your baby, you might like to consider learning baby massage as a way of deepening your connection.

Dr Tiffany Fields, Director at Touch Research Institute at the University of Miami School of Medicine, has found that a massage before bedtime is more effective than rocking at helping babies fall asleep and stay asleep. Dr Field's studies were backed up by the Warwick Medical School in the UK, whose research showed that babies who were massaged cried less, slept better and had lower levels of stress hormones than babies who didn't receive a massage.[23]

How to massage your baby

Massaging your baby is easy to do and just involves a series of slow and gentle strokes. Make sure the environment is warm and, if your baby doesn't react to oils, you can warm up some coconut oil in your hand and use it to help you massage your baby more smoothly.

Always ask permission from your baby prior to massaging her. If your baby gets agitated and seems likes she doesn't want a massage, respect this and leave the massage for another time. If at any time during the massage your child shows signs of agitation, just finish the stroke you're doing and then stop; don't force the massage on your baby.

It's good to talk your baby through the massage. Tell him what you're doing and make eye contact with your baby if possible (my son's eyes often wandered all over the place during massage, but I still cooed and told him what I was doing and he seemed to enjoy himself). Smile and have fun with your baby, as this is a wonderful bonding experience for both of you.

Massaging the feet and legs: You can use firm, gentle, slow strokes to massage the soles of your baby's feet. Continue with long strokes up your baby's leg. Hold your baby's leg under the knee and gently press it towards your baby's stomach to help expel any gas your baby might be holding. Repeat for the other leg.

Massaging the upper body: To massage your baby's upper body, make gentle strokes from your baby's shoulders to his chest. Then massage his arms from the shoulders down to the wrists in long strokes, similar to the way you massaged his legs.

Massaging the stomach: You can massage his stomach by making L-shaped movements or circular movements in very gentle, slow, clockwise circles. Just be mindful that your baby's stomach is sensitive, so stop if he shows any signs of agitation.

Massaging the face: Use your fingertips to massage your baby's face. Make gentle semi-circles, starting from the middle of your baby's forehead, moving down the outside of his face and in towards his cheeks. (I always envisage this as drawing love hearts.) You can massage your baby's scalp by making small circles with your fingertips.

Massaging the back: Turn your baby onto his stomach and use long, gentle strokes from the base of his head down to his toes.

Some other great ways to foster connection through touch include mums and bubs yoga, baby sensory classes and kangatraining. Mums and bubs yoga includes babies in some of the postures and incorporates stretching, massage and rhythmic movements. Kangatraining holds baby close to your chest as you move and dance. Baby sensory classes teaches you ways to connect and bond with your baby through different senses, including touch.

SOUND

Sound is a great way to create connections with your baby, as it soothes and relaxes your baby. There are a number of ways you can use sound to connect with your baby across the different stages.

Pregnancy

Your womb is rich with sound—the beating of your heart, the rhythmic swooshing of the placenta and the gurgling of your stomach. All of these sounds provide comfort for your baby, who will begin hearing by week eighteen of pregnancy. By week twenty-three your baby's hearing is developed enough for him to respond to external noise, and studies have shown that at the six-month mark he can move his body to the rhythm of his mother's speech.[24]

Bonding through speech

Your baby listens to your voice all day while you're in meetings, at the shops, and talking to your partner, family and friends. He gets to know your voice quite intimately, as it reaches him in a stronger form than outside noises. It provides him with a lot of comfort. Talking directly to your baby establishes your presence and communicates your love and caring to him.

When I was pregnant, I would go for a walk along the river close to my office at lunchtime. The pathway was busy with pedestrians and cyclists, but in the short bursts when no one was around I would tell my son stories about my day and talk to him about random things. I felt a bit crazy, it's a weird thing to be in public and apparently talking to yourself, but I cherished those moments.

Tell your baby stories about your day—where you're going, what you're doing, what you're eating. Tell him how excited you are to meet him and how welcome he is in your life. Read him stories. Buy or borrow your favourite children's book and read it to your baby often. Studies show that babies will recognise stories they have repeatedly heard in the womb.

My husband and I also used to read our own books to our son. It didn't really matter what the book was. It could have been a pregnancy book or a novel one of us was reading. We would read out loud in caring tones so my son would get used to our voices. We'd always combine this with touch—massage my belly, and give him a little tap and squeeze to let him know we were talking with him. We'd get a lot of joy when he'd kick and move in response.

Bonding through music

Music is another crucial way of bonding with your unborn baby. Music is thought to be pre-linguistic and contributes to your baby's foundation for language skills. Listening to music and singing songs you enjoy can provide healthy stimulation for your child's development.

Babies prefer classical music as the music has harmony and a tendency to repeat notes, which creates a lullaby effect. It also tends to mimic the mother's heart rate of sixty beats per minute. There is also non-classical music that has harmony and mimics the mother's heart rate. You can find playlists online of sixty-beats-per-minute songs in all sorts of genres that suit your tastes. Examples include Adele's 'Someone like you', Coldplay's 'Paradise', Jack Johnson's 'Better Together' and Enya's 'Sail Away'.

During pregnancy we got into the habit of tuning the radio to the twenty-four-hour classical station, and it's often our background music even now. It makes our house quite peaceful and has a strangely calming effect. Which isn't so strange, as studies have shown that people start breathing in time with the music and it helps them feel more relaxed.[25]

If classical or sixty-beats-per-minute songs aren't your thing, don't worry. Just play music that you enjoy. When you're feeling good, those feel-good hormones will pass over to your baby, making her feel calm and relaxed.

According to the experts, rock music and heavy metal is not great for unborn babies, especially as the amniotic fluid amplifies the sound.[26] They may become agitated and respond violently to the sound. That said, my husband has a major man-crush on Dave Grohl and our son was regularly exposed to music by the Foo Fighters. I used to worry about this, but now as a toddler he really enjoys bonding with his father to the sound of the Foos and gets right into the music, even singing some of the songs. It's probably best, however, not to make rock the only source of music your child hears.

You can have some fun with bonding through music. Just don't overthink it, and play music that makes you feel good. Sing along to the tunes; even if you don't think you can sing, your baby loves the sound of your voice.

When bub arrives

Your baby will love to hear the voices he or she heard while in the womb, especially her mother's and father's voices. Keep singing the songs that you sang or telling the stories you told your baby when she was in your womb.

On our son's second day in the hospital, he had his first bath. He didn't like it one bit, what with the bright lights, the chilly temperature on his bare skin and several people gawking at him. I'm sure he picked up on his parents' nervous vibes, as we were completely terrified at the thought of submerging this fragile, little person in a tub of water.

When he was placed in the water he started screaming. I'm not sure why, but I started singing 'You are my sunshine', a song I regularly sang to him in the womb. When I started to sing and my husband joined in, my son calmed right down and stopped crying. We were amazed.

The song soon became a favourite of ours to calm him with, especially when we were driving and weren't able to immediately tend to his needs.

We had a lot of fun after our son was born singing our favourite songs. I was quite adamant during pregnancy that nursery rhymes would not be the only music we listened to just because we were having a baby. So we played the music we liked, but would often slow it down to a lullaby type of rhythm. My husband sings and plays the guitar, so he'd spend time playing and crooning soft songs to our son. We purchased and were given some lullaby renditions of rock songs that have been slowed down especially for babies. It was always surreal singing along to lullaby versions of the Beatles and songs like 'Stairway to Heaven'.

Another way that sound can be used to form attachments is in the mimicking of pre-birth noises. When holding and trying to calm down an upset baby, our instincts are to rock the baby and make shushing sounds of 'shhhh, shhhh, shhhh'. It wasn't until he was several months old and I took my son to baby sensory classes that I understood what this noise represented. The shushing noise is simulating the swooshing of the placenta and provides the baby with a lot of comfort. Our intuition and innate nature knows exactly how to use sounds to bond with baby.

Baby Ears

When Juan was twelve days old, my sister told me about Baby Ears, or Dunstan Baby Language, which identifies the five universal cries that babies make before the age of twelve weeks.

Baby Ears was developed by Priscilla Dunstan, who discovered the reflexive sounds when her son was a baby. Using her unusual ability to remember audio patterns, she identified five reflexive 'pre-cries' her son made before getting worked up into a hysterical cry. Those five cries were:

Neh — I'm hungry

Owh — I'm feeling sleepy

Heh — I'm not comfortable (i.e. hot, cold, wet, in an awkward position)

Eh — I need to be burped

Eairh — I have wind or an upset tummy

Her theory has been tested with babies in different countries and cultures, and it's been recognised that babies universally use the same five reflexive and pre-emptive cries. In other words, newborn babies communicate with their parents and tell us what they need.

Learning about Baby Ears was game-changing for us. We were able to distinguish between Juan's cries and understand his needs, enabling us to quickly and calmly respond so that he didn't work himself up to a hysterical cry.

SIGHT

Sight is a sense that can be overlooked as a way to stimulate and bond with your baby. It's quite obvious and instinctual to touch and talk to your baby, but not many people think to use sight as a way to connect.

Pregnancy

Your baby's vision is developing from as early as week four. Although her eyelids stay closed until about week twenty-six, it's thought that she can respond to light and dark before this time. You can experiment by shining a light on your belly and then moving the light away. See what reaction your baby gives you. Also try bathing your belly in sunlight and see what reaction your baby gives you.

You can use sight to enhance your own emotional state, which in turn deepens your connection with your baby. If you look at scenic views, pictures, art—anything that makes you feel good—you can trigger feel-good hormones to pass to your baby. This allows your baby to mirror your emotional state. When you look at nature scenes, either in real life or pictures of nature, you can increase your feelings of calm and joy while decreasing your heart rate and blood pressure.

When bub arrives

When your baby is born, he can only see about 20-30cm, a distance that was not left to chance. That is the distance between your breast and your eyes, which helps you and your baby to bond through eye contact while breastfeeding.

If you're unable to breastfeed, you can still bond with your baby this way. Try propping your baby up on a pillow so they're only 30cm away from your face while you bottle-feed them.

Often the most stimulating object for your baby is you. From the moment of birth, and for many months afterwards, your face will provide a lot of stimulation, so try to make funny and interesting faces. It may not be practical for you to always be the entertainment, so external objects can also provide wonderful visual stimulation. In the first couple of months, high-contrast patterns, such as checkerboard patterns, will be very attractive.

Baby gyms and mobiles placed over a baby's bouncer, bassinet or cot can provide visual stimulation through the patterns, bright colours and movement. As babies can only see black, grey and white for the first few months, choose a mobile with bold patterns. From the age of about three months, one of my son's favourite activities was lying on the spare bed looking out at the branches of a tree in the neighbouring yard. Very young babies can't distinguish between colours, but they love contrast and movement. The contrast of colours between the leaves and the sky and the gentle swaying movement of the leaves in the wind kept him happily occupied. I used to joke that we needn't have bought him toys; he was happy and stimulated enough with the tree.

From around two months you can also introduce tracking games, that is, if you move toys in front of his face his eyes will follow them. You can continue this into later months, gradually introducing more brightly coloured toys and books and objects of different shapes. From about four to six months you can start introducing bub to mirrors, and he'll start noticing the smaller details on toys.

In these early days, however, don't forget that you are still the most interesting thing to bub. He will love watching and responding to your silly faces and antics.

TASTE

The sense of taste is not often associated with bonding with your baby. However, there are several ways that you can connect with your baby through the foods that you and your baby consume and these can help set up life-long habits and benefits.

Pregnancy

It's quite correct in saying that you are now eating for two. Your baby develops the capacity to taste in utero when his taste buds start to form at around seven weeks. Flavour molecules cross the placenta and the amniotic fluid acts as a conduit that allows him to taste the things that you eat. In fact, studies suggest that newborns are more accepting of flavours they have been exposed to in the womb.

When you feel good about your food, this can also be beneficial for your baby. You will release pleasure hormones which pass across the placenta so your baby can also feel pleasure from what you are eating.

You can also start setting up nutritional patterns with your baby at this early stage. If you feel good about eating fresh, wholesome food, this may help your baby associate positive feelings with nutritional choices. This may be reinforced if you combine this with sound, such as talking about your food and nutritional choices with your baby.

When bub arrives

When your baby is born, she can already sense four of the primary tastes—sweetness, bitterness, sourness and umami. At about four months, she will be able to taste saltiness. While newborns seem to dislike bitter and sour tastes, they especially love sugar solutions and glutamate (umami) that are both found in breast milk.[27]

If you're breastfeeding, it doesn't take long for the flavours from your food to reach your child. One study showed that when mothers were given garlic pills, the babies noticed the garlic odour of their breast milk and this reached a peak between one-and-a-half and three hours later.[28]

Breast milk exposes your baby to many different flavours and there is some evidence that breastfed babies are more accepting of new foods when they begin eating solids. However, it's quite possible that the effect depends on what food the mother ate while breastfeeding, so try to eat a variety of different foods.

Aside from flavours, breast milk contains over 200 different vitamins, minerals, proteins, fatty acids, amino acids, hormones, anti-inflammatory agents and other constituents such as calcium and sodium.[29] All of these nurture and nourish baby's developing body and brain and protect him against infections by providing prebiotics which stimulate the growth of beneficial bacteria and intestinal microbiota, which, in turn, seed lifelong health benefits.[30]

If you aren't able to breastfeed, your baby will still be exposed to tastes and flavours through formula, which has been created to resemble breast milk. Formula also affects long-term food preferences, although perhaps not to the full degree that breast milk does.

SMELL

According to Shawne Tassone and Kathryn Landherr, obstetricians and authors of the book *Spiritual Pregnancy*, the sense of smell lingers in the brain for longer than the other senses.[31] Odours transmit crucial information about the world. This makes smell a powerful tool for bonding with your baby.

Pregnancy

Your baby's nose develops at around eleven to fifteen weeks, and the amniotic fluid is a conduit for smell. By the end of the first trimester, baby can smell the food you're eating. So, if you are eating fragrant curries, take pleasure in the fact that your baby can also enjoy the wonderful aromatic spices.

When you smell scents that you particularly enjoy—it could be freshly ground coffee or fresh bread, beautiful flowers, your favourite perfume or even the scent of freshly cut grass—you will feel good emotionally. This pleasing feeling will cross over to your baby through hormones that communicate pleasure and happiness.

Scents can be stimulating, relaxing, invigorating and soothing. Your baby will feel whatever emotion a particular scent induces in you. If you're using essential oils during your pregnancy, refer to the aromatherapy guide in *Connect with nature*.

When bub arrives

Scent plays a significant role in bonding and communication between mother and baby. A newborn baby's smell provides motivational and emotional responses that encourage mothers to provide care functions such as breastfeeding and protection. In fact, researchers at the University of Montreal's Department of Psychology have found that mothers experience the same reward-based brain reaction when they take in the smell of a newborn baby that other people experience when smelling tempting food or taking mood-enhancing drugs.[32]

Babies are responsive to their mother's smell immediately after birth. The odour from a mother's breasts exerts a pheromone-like effect on newborns, and alert babies will do a 'breast crawl' to locate and attach themselves to their mother's nipple.[33] I have read in countless books and resources that this only happens to babies who experienced an un-medicated birth. However, my son crawled to my breast after an emergency C-section, so I know that it's possible for babies who were birthed via an intervention to do this. This may be influenced by the oxytocin that my son was exposed to during the long but relaxed labour.

Babies learn to recognise their mother's unique scent, and are able to use it to identify their mothers and distinguish them from other people. Breastfed babies become more rapidly familiarised with their mother's unique olfactory signature because they're exposed to maternal odours through the nipple-areola region while nursing.[34]

It is important in the first hours and days with your newborn that you and your partner abstain from overzealous application of perfume and cologne. Your baby needs to be able to identify your unique scent, and heavy perfume may overwhelm your natural odour and make this bonding process more difficult.

EXERCISE

1) Now that you've been through the different ways you can bond with your baby at the various stages, make a list of the connection activities in each of the five senses that you would like to try. Make note of the exercises you can do together with your partner.

2) Keep a diary of how your baby responds when you try the different bonding exercises and also keep a record of how you feel during the exercises.

3) Jot down the stories you read to bub and the songs you sing, as you can read those stories and sing those songs when he or she arrives to extend that pre-birth connection and comfort and soothe them.

PART 4:

CONNECT WITH OTHERS

'A connection is the energy that exists between people when they feel seen, heard, and valued; when they can give and receive without judgement.'

BRENE BROWN

So far on the connection compass, we have looked inwards and connected with our baby, but now it's time to connect outwardly. This section is about connecting with our partners, our families and the wider community. It's about building a support network.

Connecting with your support network focuses on strengthening the existing relationships in your life and forging new ones. It's about finding resources that will help you on your journey as a mother. It's about external connections and how to use them to give your baby the best start in life, but it will also help you stay sane and calm as you step into motherhood.

CHERISH YOUR PARTNER

These days our relationships are diverse. Many people having babies are not in traditional relationships or marriages and there are all kinds of different family arrangements, including same-sex couples, step families and single-parent families. As mentioned before, everyone's journey into parenthood is different and is influenced by their unique circumstances. So while this section relates predominantly to mothers in relationships, those of you who are preparing for parenthood as a single mother may find information here to help you connect with others.

Regardless of your circumstances, chances are when your baby arrives there will be changes in your primary relationship. You go from being lovers to being parents. From being a couple with relative freedom to being a family restricted by your baby's demands.

While it can be a struggle to adapt to these changing dynamics, maintaining a healthy relationship will help both of you in your transition to your new and evolving roles. This is an exciting time of change for both of you, and the transition will be more manageable if you can share the experience and learn and grow in a supportive environment. During pregnancy, my husband and I were really close. He was thrilled to become a father and was really supportive. We had a great relationship and were best friends. During our son's birth, we shared the journey and Leland actively participated in his support role. He was the first to see our son and I'm not sure there could have been a prouder father.

Yet, after my son was born, I turned into a lioness. I was fiercely protective of Juan and put his needs before Leland's. I suspect it was the hormones talking, but it surprised me. Coming into parenthood we had expected that Leland would be more hands-on than he was able to be. As I spent more time with Juan than Leland did, I became overbearing and critical of how Leland was taking care of our son. In hindsight, I should have let Leland find his own fatherhood rhythm and not interfered.

The change to our sex life was also unexpected. I pushed Leland away a lot, as I was exhausted and it took a while to physically recover.

The expectations we had coming into parenting were completely shattered and it took time for us to adjust. We had little time for just the two of us and genuinely missed each other. It was an unexpected transition, and I'm still learning. In fact, writing this chapter has been a lesson and exploration exercise for me.

I'd like to acknowledge the help of relationship coach Annette Baulch35 in writing the following advice on maintaining your connection with your partner throughout this transition period.

Accept change

The first and most important thing to acknowledge is that having a baby is a profound life change, for both of you, and it's going to take some adjustment. Expecting this and knowing that this is normal can make a big difference. For example:

- You may not have much time or many chances to just be the two of you for a while.
- Your partner may feel excluded if you're the one who does most of the feeding and caretaking, or if your baby soothes and calms more easily with you.
- Your glowing maternal feelings may not flow over onto your partner, and you may feel resentful when they walk out the door to the 'freedom' of work while you're at home all day caring for your baby.
- Your lifestyle might change dramatically—you may have been an active and spontaneous couple but now outings need to be planned.

Acceptance is key here. Accept that it might take an hour to get out of the house with a baby. Accept that spontaneity will be impossible for a few months until you get a handle on life with a baby.

Just acknowledging these issues and having a laugh together helps you move through them, and you will find further tips in this section and throughout this book to help you manage the change that a baby creates.

Make it a shared journey

During pregnancy, when the focus is on you and what's happening to you, it's easy to forget just how big an impact becoming a parent will have on your partner. Modern fathers are certainly becoming more directly involved in their children's care, but motherhood is still one of the most revered roles in our society. This is subtly reinforced in many different ways, from advertisements with only 'mother and baby' images to baby-care books that refer to things 'mother' can do when the child is ill. Even this book, focused on being a connected mama, reinforces this sacred role.

It's important to know this imbalance can be reflected in the husband/wife dynamic if the father role is not fully acknowledged.

For even though your partner doesn't physically carry and give birth to your baby, becoming a parent brings in life-altering changes for him, just like it has for you. These changes include:

- The added responsibility of being a provider, not only for the child but also for the mother, even if she's intending to go back to work.
- His desires/fears regarding the practical aspects of baby care and how involved he can be.
- The changed landscape of the bedroom—how to balance sexual needs with mother/child needs.
- Changes to how he sees himself as a man and father—his role versus his independence.
- Integrating the huge opening of his heart and the deep connection to this new human being.

When a couple become parents, the mother is perceived to be in the power position, but understanding this and being willing to talk about it during pregnancy helps your partner become more engaged in the process of creating and nurturing a new life. When he knows there is a place in it for him, he will pay you back in spades when your baby arrives.

There is a lot that you can do to address the power imbalance that naturally occurs when a couple has a baby. Your partner can practise the many bonding techniques suggested in this book, and there are also ways that he can feel empowered in the very early stages of parenthood, when most of the power lies with the mother.

- Find ways for your partner to support you while you breastfeed your baby, such as bringing you water, snacks or something to read. If you're bottle-feeding, your partner may take the role of feeding when they are home.

- To make sure your partner is included in caring for bub, they can have a dedicated role, like nappy changing or putting bub to bed. While it can be heartbreaking (for both of you) to listen to your baby crying when you know you can soothe her more quickly, encourage your partner to find their own groove soothing and bonding with baby.
- Remember that your baby is only completely dependent on mum for what is a fleeting time in the long run, and in a few months your partner can be more hands on.

Communicate

Keeping the lines of communication open is vital for keeping your relationship strong, and it becomes even more important when you become parents.

Make the time to talk about your post-baby expectations, fears and desires *before* your baby comes. When you do this, however, it's important that you don't expect your partner to communicate the same way that you do. These are tender topics and communication styles differ, especially between men and women. Be prepared to listen to what is being said, rather than having any expectations. Men often don't have the same language or even the social permission to express feelings the way women do. Knowing this can help you see them more clearly.

Ask open-ended questions, and focus on talking about what you fear and desire for yourself, then ask your partner about their fears and desires. Lots of people will want to give you advice, and there are zillions of articles and hundreds of books out there with helpful suggestions. Ultimately, however, it is your relationship and you need to make it work your way.

Make sure you discuss your potential parenting styles. You might not think it, but you will probably have differences in the way you want to raise your child. These differences will be reflections of the way you were brought up yourselves. Discuss the differences in your upbringing and see how this might look. Decide if you want to negotiate and present a united front or be willing to let each parent be responsible for the consequences of their individual choices.

After bub arrives, you might like to have a 'daily de-brief'. When your partner arrives home from work and has had a chance to chill out from his day, sit down together for a few minutes to discuss what's happened during the day. You may even like to structure this conversation by telling each other your high point and low point of the day. This helps you both keep up-to-date with what's happening in your lives, and you can better understand each other's emotional needs and state of mind, which can often have shifted since the morning.

You don't need words to communicate; an expression of love can be silent. Especially on days that feel like groundhog day, with the same old routine for both of you, you may wish to communicate through other means. This might include cooking each other's favourite meals, leaving notes and love letters around the house, bringing home flowers, or running a warm bath for your partner with candles and their favourite music. Sometimes just a lovely foot or back rub speaks a thousand words.

Allocate some adult time

Making the effort to maintain the vital adult-to-adult space in your relationship will potentially save you years of suffering and disconnection. This doesn't need to be a complicated arrangement, just a clearly identified space where it's just the two of you spending some time together—no baby, work or outside interests. Try to do this at least every other day, perhaps when baby is asleep. You can try sharing a meal together, chatting about your day, snuggling up together to watch your favourite TV show or making love. It doesn't matter what you do, but make sure you're not doing chores or focused on your devices while you sit next to each other. You need to be fully present and connecting as a couple.

You may wish to organise a regular date, where the two of you can get out of the house to spend some time together. It needn't even be at night; it might be breakfast or even a run if that was something you used to enjoy together before bub arrived. Make the most of your babysitting options, and offer to look after your friends' babies in return.

Bringing your sexy back

You should also discuss post-baby sex while you're pregnant. Sex during pregnancy can be really fulfilling and some women say it's the best sex of their lives. But sex is going to look a little different for a while after your baby arrives. For a time you'll be so tired or frazzled (or both), you won't even want to think about it, and that's okay. The main thing is to talk about it and have a plan; otherwise, there is the potential for your baby to take over the place where the sex used to be. This is not good for your relationship in the long term and is the quickest way to drive a wedge between you and your partner.

Talk with your partner about:
- How sex is important to you and how, ultimately, you do want it to be a part of your relationship.
- How there will initially be a time when you're just not up for it, due to your hormones rebalancing themselves, sleep deprivation, healing episiotomy scars and feeding issues. Know that this is normal.
- How things like doing the dishes, tidying up, bathing the baby or answering the phone to your mother may become a type of foreplay. Explain how being freed from draining activities like cleaning, without having to ask, can be very attractive to a woman.

Once you've adjusted to your new routine and you're physically recovering, you might like to explore some of the following ideas:

- Understand that your body may feel different post-baby, so just explore it without judgement. You may feel different too— more comfortable, powerful or tentative. However you feel, know that your sexy, desirable woman is still there, and she just needs time to come out. Your partner knows this and is likely to be very willing to support you.
- Feeling sexual is about feeling connected to your sense of self. Finding ways for you to regain your sense of who you are will help nurture this part of you. Identify what it is that most makes you feel like you and find ways to fit these experiences into your life—for example, going for a walk or run, meditating, having coffee with your girlfriends, taking time to shop for yourself, doing your hobby or having a few hours at a spa.
- Have your partner remind you that you're a sexual being by helping you get back into your sexual feelings. For example, stroking or kissing the back of your neck or inner arms, massaging your feet, hugging you from behind (without touching breasts) and connecting your hearts. This only works when you don't have an agenda to turn it into instant sex. Think about the bigger picture of maintaining long-term connection and just enjoy the moment.
- Try just lying together with your hand resting on his penis and his hand resting on your heart, maybe as you go to sleep. This validates the sexual connection between you.
- Know that you may be initially more interested in 'connecting' sex—going slower, relaxing, breathing more and taking your time—than highly erotic, hot and heavy 'performance' sex. This may be more difficult with a baby, but you can try to time sex to coincide with baby's nap times.
- Understand that, in this place, arousal can come before desire. This means that actually creating some pleasure through touch (or feeling your partner's pleasure) can assist your own desire for making love to arise.

- Practice 'Daily Devotion'—a tantric practice that is about connection rather than outcome. There is no foreplay and no orgasm. Take up a side-by-side or scissors position. Use just enough lubrication to enable penetration, and then engage in slow or no movement, just maintain connection for ten to ten minutes. Relax, breathe and feel what is, then hug to complete. This is a great way to re-establish the sexual energy between you. If daily is unrealistic with a baby, there is benefit in practising as often as possible.
- Support your man in his desire to self-pleasure by not making him wrong for it. Instead think of him keeping his love energy connection alive to share with you when you are ready to return to lovemaking.

What to do if issues arise

Challenges occur in all relationships, and with a healthy, loving connection these can generally be resolved with some goodwill, especially if the desire to feel connected and at ease with each other is stronger than the desire to prolong the hurt. However, if any of the following red flags occur on a regular basis, then it is time to seek some professional help:

- You and/or your partner are consistently feeling flat, stuck or overwhelmed and nothing seems to help.
- You and/or your partner are losing interest in your baby or find yourselves getting angry with them.
- You're having frequent arguments where you just blame or criticise each other, or you're hardly talking at all, and things never get resolved.
- It feels like you and/or your partner are just not putting the effort into your relationship to connect, to talk, to spend time together.

- Differences between you have become barriers. For example, you can't make decisions about childcare, finances, your social life and so on.
- It's hard to find empathy or compassion for each other, and the care factor just doesn't seem to be there.
- You are unable to resolve issues between you in the bedroom.
- You start feeling unsafe in your relationship.

If you have a good relationship with your doctor and/or child health nurse, this might be a good place to start looking for help. If you feel you need counselling, then there are national associations and directories where you can find a counsellor in your local area. Most people are daunted at the thought of couples counselling and instead seek individual counselling as a less confronting option. This may provide a short-term boost, but counselling for both of you reaps greater rewards—your partner's agreement to have counselling can be proof they care. Couples counselling focuses on the relationship and provides a safe place where both of you get equal time, attention and understanding.

FOSTER HARMONY WITH SIBLINGS

I have only one child but I do often wonder how the transition will go for Juan when he has a sibling. It's something I am always curious about when my sisters or friends have another baby—how do they maintain harmony, especially with the elder child who, until now, has been the centre of mum and dad's universe? Motherhood is always evolving and there is a constant need to learn new skills and adapt.

The following strategies were adapted from materials by the Australian parenting website RaisingChildren.net.au[36] and also from Dr Laura Markham, clinical psychologist, author and creator of AhaParenting.com.[37]

Preparing your child for a new baby

- Involve your child in the bonding exercises included in this book. For example, ask them to talk and sing to baby, let them touch your belly and gently 'play' with baby. If possible, have them listen to baby's heartbeat at a prenatal care visit.
- Let them help you prepare for the practical aspect of having a new baby by doing things such as picking out clothes, toys and furniture. You may like to invite them to paint some little canvases for baby's nursery.
- You might also wish to ask them for name options. My nephew named his little brother—my sister asked him for options and he came up with the perfect name.
- Talk to your child about how every member of the family has a special role and that they will be the big sister or brother, which is a wonderful contribution to the family.

When you're having bub

- When baby arrives, you may want your older child to come and see you in the hospital before other visitors arrive. Let them sit and hold the baby, helping them support bub's head. According to bonding expert Dr Lawrence Aber, babies' heads give off pheromones that encourage us to fall in love and begin to feel protective. Allow your child to snuggle into baby to deepen their attachment and bond.
- If appropriate, ask visitors to bring a small gift for the older child so they can feel like there is indeed something to celebrate. Also consider a special gift from bub to their big sister or brother.

Settling in as a family

- When you come home, be sensitive to the feelings of your older children, who may think that you're giving all the attention to bub. Listen and give them lots of attention to show that you're still there for them and help them feel secure. Even though you'll be very busy with your baby, try to spend some one-on-one time with your older child.
- Spending special time with your older children while you tend to your baby's needs is a wonderful way to strengthen the bond between your child and your partner or other family members.
- See what elements of baby care your child can help you with. Maybe they can help with bath time, or take part in massage by rubbing oil on your baby's legs.
- When breastfeeding, it can help to have a box of goodies and toys beside you to help you manage your older child if they want to be close to you and bub. You can read them a story or they can draw a picture or play with a toy. You may wish to put on your child's favourite music so you can sing together. Your bub will love that too.

CHERISH YOUR COMMUNITY

There is a wonderful African proverb that says, 'It takes a village to raise a child'. I believe it should have rounded off with, 'It also takes a village to raise a mother."

In traditional cultures, the responsibility for raising a child ultimately rests with the parents, but grandparents have a considerable influence, the extended family gets involved, and the community also plays a role. This is very different from the typical experience of a working western mother who is used to managing on her own, may have no family nearby to help her, and may not know what resources are available in her local community. This is a shame, because after spending six years living in Asia at different times and in different countries, I have observed how valuable the village can be in raising children and supporting mothers.

I've spent time in remote villages in Nepal, where women don't have the information and resources available to them that we have in the West. Electricity was a luxury, and water had to be collected by hiking to the nearest communal pump. Internet and mobile communication wasn't on tap like it is for us. Yet the mothers weren't anxious or isolated because they were surrounded by family and friends, wise women and respected elders who passed on their valuable knowledge, traditions and remedies.

Your main priority as a new mother is to bond and fall in love with your baby. Your village or support network can help alleviate the burden of tasks that otherwise might distract you from that important role. This can be hard for professional women who are used to being strong and independent, and who may have lost touch with their community at a grassroots level. But remember that it's not a weakness to ask for help, and it's okay to let people do things for you if that's what you want or need.

While your intuition will help with your transition to motherhood, the people and resources in your village can help with many of the practical aspects of new motherhood, such as how to change a nappy, how to turn a huge piece of material into a secure sling for your baby, or how to install a car seat. If you're having issues breastfeeding, there are lactation consultants available to support you.

Your village can help you with less tangible matters too, such as your emotional needs and forming meaningful friendships and relationships. Loneliness and isolation are an often unexpected part of early motherhood, so having a village that can help you maintain connection and a sense of self is of vital importance.

If you're unsure about how to interact with your child, there are classes like infant massage and baby sensory classes that can help with that. Having a village around you can also help to validate the job you're doing as a mother. This is something that mothers tell me all the time and it's something I felt too. In our professions, we're used to getting feedback and validation on a daily basis. Suddenly, in motherhood, that validation from respected peers isn't as forthcoming. Your baby is dependent on you and your partner, and his or her constant demands can make you question yourself and your decisions. Having networks you trust can help you find validation and positive feedback in your new role. This, in turn, helps you build self-esteem and confidence.

We're living in a society where there is an endless amount of help around us. All we need to do is look for it and be discerning in our selection.

Don't let the village find you

You've probably heard the 'village' proverb before, but some of you may have also seen the bumper sticker that says, 'I've seen the village and I don't want it raising my children'.

Obviously, it's sarcastic, and is intended to have a go at modern society and education systems in particular. And there's some truth to it. There are people and influences out there that may not be beneficial for either you or your child. So that you can be prepared, let's look at some of those.

There is the danger that well-meaning people may step in and provide advice that you didn't want or ask for. For example, friends, strangers or even Great-Aunty Sally may volunteer information about how you should be settling your bub into feeding or sleeping routines, and this may throw you off kilter. You may be led down a road that you didn't wish to go down and it may take more effort to get back on track than if you had put the effort in up-front not to falter.

You should also be discerning about the online help you seek out. Trust me, when your baby is vomiting or has a high temperature at 3am, grabbing your iPad and Googling a diagnosis can be a sure-fire recipe for stress and anxiety. I learnt that the hard way, but eventually found one or two sites that I respected and would consult those first for advice. For example, Ask Dr Sears resonated with my preference for attachment parenting. If I was feeling uneasy, I would ring 13HEALTH and get reassurance from a nurse. In other instances, my husband and I simply trusted our instincts, bundled up our son and drove him to the hospital.

I'm also quite discerning about using social media for parenting advice. Social media can be really addictive for new mothers. New mothers often feel isolated and lonely, so to have a sense of connection many women reach out to friends and networks on Facebook, Instagram and other social media. It's quite addictive because not only can you connect with the outside world, you can also often find the validation you may be seeking.

Notwithstanding the security issues around posting on the Internet about your child and family, when you join closed parenting groups on Facebook, be selective. Some may be life-savers and provide you with rich connections that can set up lifetime friendships. Others may be a drain on your energy and can do more harm than good. If you want to join Facebook groups, you'll find a huge variety out there. There are groups that cater for specific interests, ones that cover a geographical region, and others that are aimed at supporting a particular type of parent, such as single parents or parents of twins. Whatever your needs, interests and circumstances, there will be something out there that will resonate with you.

There is a lot of value in mums supporting other mums. Just be mindful that it can be a case of strangers giving you advice when they don't know your particular circumstances, beliefs and worldview. So, take all advice you receive (and even the advice that you give) within that frame of reference. In the early days, it's beneficial to be surrounded with support, nurturing and love, so find networks that will provide you with that.

Find your own village

Now that I've warned you about some of the dangers that might lurk in the village, let's look at a way of pro-actively creating a village—one that you know is right for you. There is no one-size-fits-all approach to parenting. Each of us needs to forge out our own support network that suits our family circumstances, our baby, our confidence levels, our lifestyle and our parenting preferences.

You can start building your village when you're pregnant, and it's great to have a structure in place that you can use for support should you need it. However, it's good to be mindful that things do change when you have a baby—your mindset can change, you might find you need more support, or you might need less support as you become more experienced as a mother. It's a good idea to put a structure in place, but be open enough to let that support change and flow according to your current needs. That enables a wonderful blend of both your feminine and masculine energies and allows balance.

When considering the village you want to gather around you, have a think about the different groups of people in your life, your interests and your family dynamic.

EXERCISE

1) Get out your trusty journal and jot down notes as you work through this activity. You may also wish to use an Excel spreadsheet for recording some of this information, as your circumstances may change as your pregnancy/motherhood journey progresses.

2) Make a list of a 'village' you may want to pull together. To help I've put together a number of questions that might help you explore the types of support you think you may like or need:
   - Think about the role that you'd like your partner to play in supporting the family. Can he (or she) pick up more of the household chores, can they do some of the midnight feeds, or can they wake up early with the baby so you can sleep in?

- Do you have any family that you can call on for support? Perhaps they live close by. If not, you may want to organise for them to visit you, or vice versa.
- Do you have friends who are also pregnant or have recently had children? That way you can embark on this new journey with people you already know and hold dear.
- Seek out the 'wise women' who can guide you. Are there any role models that you'd like to emulate as you become a mother? For example, this could be your mother, sisters, aunties, cousins, friends or even a family friend.
- What kind of birth would you like to have? Can you do a course to prepare or would you like to hire a doula (birth coach) to accompany you on the journey? Can you actively seek the experiences of people who had the birth you hope to have, so you can set a new norm/belief structure about childbirth? If you do a course, can you keep in touch with some of the parents and share the experience across pregnancy, birth and motherhood?
- How do you hope to nourish your baby when she's born—are you hoping to breastfeed? Are there people you can ask for advice, like lactation consultants or a community focused on breastfeeding? Can you connect with them before having your baby? This way you will have people you know you can trust ready to call on if you need help later on.
- When your baby is born, can your hospital or community nurse refer you to a local mothers' group?
- Do you have a family doctor and pharmacist that you particularly like and whose advice you can trust for bub's first few months?
- Would you benefit from seeing an energy practitioner who can help you prepare for your baby's birth and help you find balance after your baby arrives? This might include

practitioners that perform emotional release, reiki, acupuncture, ka huna massage and so on.

- Is there a particular parenting style that speaks to you? For example, attachment parenting really spoke to me, and I sought both a community as well as a trusted source of information to refer to when I needed help.

- What activities for babies are available in your local area? I found that meeting mums that were only a walk or short drive away made a huge difference in my happiness and sanity levels as a new mama.

- Think back to Connecting with you. What interests excite you and give you joy? Can you find mothers' groups or playgroups that meet regularly that share your interests? (www.meetup.org has groups that cover all sorts of interests. If you can't find a group to cover your particular interests, you can organise one.)

- Who in your current group of friends or circle of influence will be able to support you in other ways? For example, your girlfriends without babies may help you keep in touch with outside interests and help encourage some 'me time'.

- Can you arrange catch-ups with your colleagues when your baby arrives to keep you current and in touch with work?

3) Now that you have a rough list of your 'village' go through and see what actions you can do today to start building your village.

For example, you may wish to contact the local breastfeeding support group, or you may make a list of friends who are pregnant that you can catch up with.

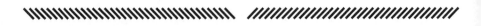

The list you have just developed will form the basis of your village and, therefore, you may wish to keep this information somewhere readily available as you go through your motherhood journey. This will become a helpful ready reference you can draw upon during difficult moments to allow you the support you need at the time.

When gathering your community around you, find people who speak to your heart. Find people who you feel will support you, who are accepting and who won't see this time as a competition. Your transition to motherhood is a sacred rite of passage, a beautiful and special time. So gather a village you truly connect with and who you truly wish to walk the path beside you.

You may get carried away trying to find your village, with Excel spreadsheets, hours of research online and endless to-do lists. Or you may think you're too independent to find people to help you. But you don't need to be super-organised to find a village, nor do you need to force it. You'll be pleasantly surprised to discover how the right help will manifest for you.

The story of how I found my village will help explain what I mean.

How I found my village

When I was a new mother, I'd often think about my situation compared with that of my friends in Nepal or India or the Philippines. In many ways I was more connected—to conveniences, to support services, to medical facilities, to information, to online friends. However, I was also a lot more isolated. My parents lived a three-hour drive away and my in-laws lived in three different countries, with the closest an eight-hour flight away. I had one or two friends who had babies a few months older than my son. Other than that, it was really just me, my husband and our baby.

I realised that I needed and wanted a village around me, but it would have to be a village that I chose and put together myself.

In thinking about my village, I realise that I cast the net wide.

Our family has been a wonderful pillar—always available, always there to listen, even though they're hundreds of kilometres away. Before Juan was born, I asked my mother, aunties and sisters for advice, which I kept for many months on a corkboard to give me strength in the early days.

When we decided to do a hypnobirthing course mid-way through our pregnancy, we found HypnoBirthing Australia and never looked back. A support framework and network opened up to us and empowered us in ways we wouldn't have thought possible.

Just prior to Juan's birth, we attended a breastfeeding course with the Australian Breastfeeding Association (ABA). We had a great morning and found it so valuable that after our son was born we returned the favour by doing the breastfeeding demonstration at the following course. I really valued my membership with ABA and, while I didn't take full advantage of it, I was always comforted knowing they were there if I needed them.

We used midwifery care during pregnancy through the Royal Brisbane and Women's Hospital's Birth Centre. We formed a lovely bond with our midwife and still keep in touch.

We had maternity photos taken just before my son was born, and newborn photos just days after he arrived. We formed a wonderful relationship with our photographer and her husband and they have been a terrific support, especially in the early days.

We were also fortunate to find a wonderful family doctor who was a blessing during pregnancy and my son's early days. I went through several doctors until, finally, I found someone I was really comfortable with and trusted. He was patient and took time to teach me what to look out for, what to be concerned about, and what not to be concerned about. He never judged or roused on me if I was a bit over-cautious (or under-cautious in some instances) and always seemed pleased to see how we were progressing. The local pharmacist was the same. She seemed to really connect with us and would often come down to the shop floor to give me some advice or just have a chat.

I'm usually one to go against the grain, and that happened with mothers' groups. Most people told me how valuable mothers' groups were, but I did hear a couple of horror stories along the way. To be honest, I was a bit confused by the concept of it. I didn't want to be put together with a group of people and find the only thing we had in common was a baby and a postcode. I wanted to share this experience with people who had mutual interests. Specifically, I wanted to be able to talk about current affairs, because my greatest fear when I was pregnant was that I'd lose interest in the outside world after Juan was born.

This is why, even though I acknowledge how valuable they are, I didn't join a local mothers' group. Instead, I sought the support of friends who were having children around the same time. I also searched groups online that shared my specific interests and reached out to them. To this day, I'm immensely grateful and close with some of the mums and families I met through those forums.

However, I don't want you to think you *have* to find kindred mother spirits through careful and targeted research. I randomly met my two best mama friends at our local library's baby rhyme time. We got chatting, went for a coffee, and have become as close as sisters. Last Christmas, we decided to spend our Christmas Day together. Our sons are each other's best friends. Our husbands have become friends in their own right. We have been through many highs and lows together, but the thing I love the most is that we can just be ourselves around each other. No hiding, no pretences. We can be vulnerable; we can be strong. We can just be.

And then there is our son's carer and early childhood educator. We use family day care and are absolutely thrilled with the lady who looks after our son. She's kind and motherly (to all of us), and in terms of our moral beliefs, we just connect.

I wouldn't expect anyone else's community to be the same as mine. Everyone forges their own community and the best ones emerge when the community is actively sought. Sometimes our village may be just as we expect it to be, but other times it may be surprising. You just have to be open to possibilities.

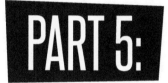

PART 5:

CONNECT WITH NATURE

'I go to nature to be soothed and healed, to have my senses be put in order.'

JOHN BURROUGHS

U p to this point, the connection compass has been helping you connect with people—with yourself, your baby, your partner, your family and the wider community. But at the final point on the connection compass, we learn how to connect with nature.

Although many of us are now urban or suburban dwellers, for ninety-nine per cent of our evolutionary history we have lived in nature. Our physiological and emotional development is still attached to nature. We belong to nature. In fact, we *are* nature and our reproductive cycles reflect this.

The cycle of conception, pregnancy and birth is the highest form of creation. It is also predominantly natural and spontaneous, with much of the process being beyond our control. This idea can be a challenge for those of us who are used to being in control of our lives.

Nature teaches

The word for nature in Chinese is *zìrán*—which translates as 'that which happens of itself'.

If you have a garden, you understand the spontaneity of nature. As much as you may weed and trim your garden, new sprouts emerge constantly and often in unexpected places. Nature is something we can't conquer and gardeners know it's a whole lot easier if we work *with* nature rather than *against* it.

Given that we're natural beings, our emotions are the same—it's easier when we work *with* them rather than fight *against* them. It's the same with the commencement of labour; unless you receive help from medical professionals, your baby will spontaneously decide when they want to enter the world. Again, with giving birth, when you work

105

with how nature designed your body to birth, the process is calmer and a great deal less painful.

It helps us immensely to understand that our baby's development, the labour and the act of birth, along with the emotions that come with it, are *zìrán*. Having an awareness of the ever-changing cycles involved in pregnancy, birth and the post-partum period can help us in our motherhood transition. The challenges thrown at us and our emotional states are temporary, and a nice mantra to keep in mind in difficult times is: 'This too shall pass'.

Nature not only teaches us that everything shall pass, but also teaches us how to nurture growth.

Nature is embodied in the feminine as a mother figure—Mother Nature—who is inherently healing and nurturing. When we enter motherhood, being nurtured by Mother Nature allows us to learn how to be nurturers ourselves. Mother Nature is a wonderful teacher of 'flowing' during our new states of pregnancy, childbirth and motherhood, and the more we can be present and allowing, the healthier our emotions and bodies will be. This helps us to give our precious baby the best start in life that we can, and also gives us the strength and resilience to cope with the ongoing changes brought about by motherhood.

But, unfortunately, many of us have become disconnected from nature. Living and working in artificial environments denies us the exposure to the healing properties of nature. Our mind, body and soul are screaming for connection with nature, even if our conscious mind doesn't understand this. Those of us who are urban dwellers are likely to have a deficit of nature unless we actively seek it out.

Luckily, however, it's easy to connect with Mother Nature and learn her valuable lessons. All we need to do is simply be in nature. There is no need to *try*; you just need to *be*. Literally, just spending time in nature teaches us to nurture, brings forth our feminine energy and heals us emotionally and physically.

This section will provide you with easy strategies to rediscover nature, which will provide you with restorative and healing energy that helps you step into your own mother role.

For those of you who are already strongly connected to nature, this section will deepen your connection and provide you with even greater grounding and healing to take into motherhood and share with your baby.

Nature heals

A national survey conducted in Ireland concerning the health of working women during pregnancy showed that stress or anxiety caused the greatest impact on their health, especially for those in managerial or administrative positions. This was followed by emotional health problems, fatigue, tiredness and exhaustion.[38] These are health issues that are not easily remedied with drugs or western medicine, but can be treated effectively by more natural means.

Nature is a tremendous healer if we connect with its restorative properties. Society has known this through the ages and passed down various remedies and techniques—essential oils and natural balms, healing foods, herbs and teas, natural rites and ceremonies—from generation to generation. In recent times, scientific and medical studies have begun to provide proof that backs up these ancient remedies.

Ancient cultures know that nurturing and easing the burden of mothers-to-be and new mothers will relieve stress for both them and their baby, which will be beneficial for emotional and physical health. Science tells us that a mother's hormones cross the placenta and enter her baby's blood supply. The higher the cortisol (stress hormone) level in the mother's blood, the greater the cortisol level in baby's amniotic fluid.[39] What ancient wisdom and present-day science both tell us is that if we can eliminate our stresses and unnecessary fatigue, we won't pass those hormones across to our babies.

Spending time in nature is a great way to reduce stress and increase our overall well-being. It helps lower our cortisol level, which allows us to be in optimal health and, in turn, this helps our bodies cope with the profound and miraculous changes involved in growing and supporting a baby. Our emotional resilience and happiness is also increased when our immune system is healthy and our stress levels are low. There are some great examples of how nature has proven to be beneficial in healing our minds and body, which I will now explore.

Stephen Kaplan, a psychologist at the University of Michigan, developed a theory in the 1980s called the Attention Restoration Theory, which states that nature can be used to restore the fatigue caused by voluntary or directed attention. Voluntary or directed attention is the attention we give to all the things that aren't essential but, nonetheless, are important enough to make us want to deal with them.

As professionals, directed attention is part and parcel of our work. There is the constant barrage of emails, the side project that has been handed to us, the participation on a committee that takes our focus away from our primary role, and so the list goes on.

We become fatigued and irritated by the pressure of all these tasks and take this stress with us into other areas of our lives, which include our pregnancy and relationships.

What can help, according to Kaplan, is sleep and spending time in nature. Outside in nature, we're free to focus our attention on any one of her minute but amazing spectacles—the wandering flight of a butterfly, a pair of frolicking finches, or the sound of leaves rustling in the breeze. The unwinding of our mind begins even as we're watching a beautiful sunset or observing a formation of ducks fly overhead.

This works because the type of attention we use to focus on nature requires little energy and it allows our mind to wander to other things. In essence, it's a form of unwinding, letting the mind drift and daydream and enter a state of allowing all the good stuff we want in our life.

Forest medicine is another tangible example of how nature can be a calming, rejuvenating and restorative force. Spending time in wild and natural areas has preventive health benefits such as increasing energy levels, promoting better sleep, reducing stress and providing an improved mood. Much of the research comes out of Japan, where Yoshifumi Miyazaki, Japan's leading scholar on forest medicine, has quantified the impact forest therapy can have on people. *Shinrin yoku*, or 'taking in the forest atmosphere or forest bathing', is the experience of being in nature, particularly walking among trees. It creates neuro-psychological effects through changes in the nervous system. Experiencing the sensory elements of nature, in particular forests, provides many benefits:

- Smelling the natural odours sparks physiological changes such as relaxation and comfort.
- Listening to the sounds of running streams instils calm.
- Observing the beauty of forest scenes comforts and soothes.
- Breathing phytocites, the volatile organic compounds that plants emit to protect themselves from bacteria, fungi and insects, boosts the immune system.[40]

The longer the time spent in nature, the greater the health benefits, but there are benefits to be had in just a twenty-minute walk. Interestingly, studies show that some of these benefits may last up to seven days after exposure.

Nature is also wonderful for babies and little children; they really respond to nature and all the sensations that it provides. Miyazaki's studies have shown that when your baby is born, taking her for a walk in the forest will have a calming effect on her. Spending time together in nature will help you to bond, as you both absorb the calming influences.

The beauty of healing through nature is its sheer simplicity and availability. You don't have to go very far to be in nature. While getting out into forests on a regular basis is advisable, it's possible to connect with nature just by sitting on a bench in a park or garden for twenty minutes. Most cities have areas of bushland and waterways, all of which are nature-rich and restorative. Even looking up at the night sky—watching the stars, the moon and the drifting of clouds—is an act of connecting with nature.

COMING TO YOUR SENSES

Connecting with nature comes naturally, and simply immersing your whole being in a natural environment is wonderfully healing. But there are also ways of bringing nature into your life that you may not have thought of, and which involve using each of your five senses in a specific way.

Touch
Give that tree a little cuddle

I fully acknowledge that tree hugging has a bad rap. It's seen as something hippies do. I will confess, however, that I don't mind a bit of a cuddle with a tree.

My most memorable tree-hugging experience was trying to wrap my arms around the world's largest living organism—the mighty sequoia (red wood) tree in Muir Woods in California. At the time, I was pregnant, and it seems I've well and truly passed the tree-hugging gene onto my son. From the time he was just a few weeks old, I would run his hands along the bark of trees and now he needs no encouragement to touch trees and wrap his arms around them.

Now we have that confession out of the way, let's talk about the scientific evidence behind the benefits of tree hugging. Author Matthew Silverstone used the results of scientifically validated studies in his book *Blinded by Science* to show the health benefits of touching trees.[41]

Silverstone explains that, at its core, every atom vibrates. This means that every object made of atoms also vibrates, but at different frequencies. Trees have unique vibrational patterns that cause positive changes in our biological behaviours when we touch them. They align any mismatches in our vibration to the tree's vibration, bringing about harmony in our being.

Oxytocin, the so-called love hormone that is responsible for feelings of calm and emotional bonding, is released when we give out hugs. If you hug a tree while pregnant, this will help you bond with bub. Other hormones such as serotonin and dopamine, which are directly linked with making you happier, are also released.

If your pregnant belly is in the way of a good tree hug, you can place your hands on the bark of the tree for healing effects.

Take off your shoes and get grounded

A person is grounded when they're energetically in contact with their body, which, in turn, puts them in contact with the earth, hence the term 'grounded'. We know when we're not grounded; it's harder to cope with the little things and we're easily thrown off balance. Being grounded, in contrast, is a feeling of solidity, presence and increased awareness. It allows you to feel free and fluid at the same time as feeling stable, as you accept your current reality and go with it. This is a wonderful skill to bring into your motherhood journey at a time when your whole world has been thrown upside down.

So how do we become more grounded?

Given my tendency is to live in my mind, I spend a lot of time and effort grounding myself. Breathing exercises, qigong, yoga and other techniques that align masculine and feminine energies are all instrumental for grounding. However, a really simple way to become more grounded is to spend time in nature.

The earth contains negatively charged ions, which are created when it's struck by lightning and showered with electrons as a result of solar activities. When our bare skin connects with the earth, we absorb these electrons into our body. This helps to neutralise free radicals caused by positively charged ions absorbed from pollution, air conditioning, WIFI and radio frequencies, and our growing collection of electronic devices.

Walking barefoot on the earth or on materials that come from the earth (with the exception of wood) allows the healing negative charges to freely flow into our bodies. Scientific studies have linked bare skin contact with a reduction of inflammation, an enhanced immune system, heightened clarity and reduced production of cortisol.[42]

You don't have to spend a lot of time grounding with nature; just five minutes a day will give you tremendous benefits. Try the following:

- Hang the washing on the line barefoot.
- Find a green patch in the city during your lunchbreak, kick off your shoes and connect your feet with the earth.
- Walk barefoot in the backyard or visit a local park.

Going barefoot on grass feels great, but there are other ways to increase the negative ions in your environment. Natural elements such as water and salt also emit negatively charged ions. Spending time near a waterfall, or walking along the beach near the salt water and crashing waves are wonderful ways to absorb negative ions.

Being in the water also helps; it is not only a fabulous exercise in grounding our energy, but also helps us get out of our heads and into our bodies.

Become a water mother

Pregnancy is a great time to connect with water. Our first experience in life was in our mother's water-filled womb. We are, in turn, creating and nurturing new life in our water-based amniotic sac. It makes sense to spend as much time as possible in water during this phase of our life.

Water has incredible therapeutic benefits during pregnancy, childbirth and post-partum. Women can find comfort, relaxation and vitality through spending time in aquatic environments, particularly those found in nature.

When submerged in water, your body becomes lighter and more buoyant. Your pregnant uterus, which is largely made up of water, tends to make floating easier. You experience only fifteen per cent of the effects of gravity, which lessens the impact on joints and reduces muscular pressure and the strain of the growing pregnant body. This allows for greater mobility than other forms of land-based activity as your pregnancy progresses. Furthermore, when submerged in water, the body requires less oxygen, which means more of the body's resources go to healing and regeneration of cells.[43]

This makes swimming and other water-based exercise (such as prenatal aqua classes) fantastic choices during your pregnancy. The benefits include working the cardiovascular system, temporary relief of swelling in wrists, hands and ankles, and support for breasts.

Spending time in water at swimming pools, natural pools and the beach also helps to cool down pregnant bodies on hot summer days.

Many maternity wards provide warm water baths for women in labour. Warm water can help ease pain as it increases the body's production of endorphins and is also believed to speed up labour. This is likely due to enhanced relaxation and reduced stress for mother and baby, as well as reduced pressure on the body which, in turn, allows for increased mobility.

Birthing in water allows both the mother and baby to work with the buoyancy of water and natural gravitational pull, which opens up the mother's pelvis and allows baby to descend more readily.[44] The theory behind water birth is that baby will have a less confronting experience as they transition from one water-based environment to another. However, it's always best to discuss the benefits and risks with your care provider.

Post-partum, both you and your baby can benefit from the healing qualities of water. You can bond as a family in water through structured activities such as baby swimming lessons, or just spend time together playing in natural environments such as the beach and parks. Older babies love splashing in water, and there is nothing more heart-warming than seeing your baby's smiles and happiness as they engage with nature.

Go low and get close with the earth

Squatting is another way to connect with nature. Energy movement practices such as yoga and qigong view squatting as a position that allows a deeper connection with the earth. It opens the sacrum and spine and places the womb directly over the earth, which grounds and opens the base chakra while drawing the earth's energy into the body.

Squatting is increasingly used during birth preparations as it's an optimal position for labour and delivery. It works with gravity and shortens the length of the birth canal. Studies also suggest that squatting during birth may decrease the likelihood of medical intervention.

I regularly squat in nature to connect and align my feminine energy with the earth's energy. I don't do this in any particularly special or thoughtful way; it's mainly done while weeding my garden. See if you can find ways to practice squatting during your pregnancy—it will help you easily adopt this position during labour as well as foster a womb connection with nature. If you find it difficult to achieve, make sure you're squatting with your feet flat on the ground and not on your tiptoes, which strains the calf muscles. If you are heavily pregnant, it's a good idea to have something or someone close-by to help you balance and come upright afterwards.

Feel free to feel nature

Engaging with the tactile elements of nature releases feel-good hormones. For example, feeling the warm tickle of the sun's rays on your skin (in moderation of course) has been proven to reduce depression and also boosts your immune system.

In my own experience, touching elements of nature has always been highly soothing for me. My favourite ways to touch nature include:

- Running my fingers through the fine sand on a beach.
- Picking a flower and playing with its petals or making flower necklaces.
- Sitting and playing with grass.

These moments of touching nature are especially powerful if those moments are combined with catching up with friends or spending time with family. Why not organise a picnic or a trip to the beach as a regular outing?

Whatever you enjoy doing that involves experiencing the tactile side of nature, do more of it.

Sight

The views in nature often take my breath away. I remember times in my life when I have been moved to tears by the spectacular views provided by nature: taking in the thousand-year-old rice paddies in the northern Philippines; snorkelling in the Great Barrier Reef and seeing the range of colour and life underwater; observing the majestic rush of water at Victoria Falls; and seeing the morning sun's rays hit the first peak of the snow-capped mountains in the Himalaya.

Observing views in nature is awe-inspiring. However, it's also been proven to decrease heart rate and blood pressure and increase feelings of calmness and joy.[45]

The examples I've given are extreme, and when you're several months pregnant or have a newborn baby it's unlikely that you'll be heading off to Zimbabwe to check out Victoria Falls. Luckily, natural views are accessible to the majority of us, whether it's a forest, a beach, a river, a look-out, a dam or a waterfall. In fact, you don't even need to be in nature for the healing effects to take place. Just looking at pictures of nature can help you feel happier and increase your cognitive performance. You may consider a visit to an art gallery, where the artworks—sculptures, photographs and paintings of nature—can be especially profound.

Spending time gazing at nature can also help with the condition known as 'baby brain' that many pregnant women and new mothers experience. More vivid than the computer screens we spend a lot of time in front of, the range and contrast of colours in nature forces our brains to work harder to process it all. This helps to increase the activity in the brain and develops our neural pathways.[46] In other words, looking at nature may help mothers get back to our pre-baby brain days and deepen our memory recall.

Smell

Smell has commonly been associated with instinct and emotion, and has a greater influence on physiological change than other senses. The aromas of nature have long been used for healing. Throughout the ages people have extracted oils from grasses, seeds, flower petals, buds, barks, wood, stems, leaves and roots and used them in aromatherapy. These scents can soothe your mind and uplift and balance your mental and emotional state. This can be useful for easing discomforts during the child-birthing year.

Aromatherapy for your child-birthing year

Pregnancy

You should exercise caution when using essential oils during pregnancy and seek the advice of your care provider. Essential oils are highly concentrated substances extracted from plants; some can be harmful for your baby or have too strong an impact on a particular organ or system of the body. Oils should be avoided during the first trimester and then used sparingly for the rest of your pregnancy. During pregnancy you should avoid oils that are cleansing or stimulating, and instead use oils that are relaxing and calming.

Lavender oil can reduce anxiety and relieve stress and can be used in a diffuser or oil burner, or in a misting spray. Lavender can also be used to relieve headaches by mixing half the normal dosage with a carrier oil and massaging it into the temples. This is quite handy when you're avoiding conventional pain relievers during pregnancy.

Ginger and sweet orange oil inhaled from a tissue can relieve nausea and morning sickness. To relieve swelling, you can soak your hands and feet in a bath mixed with a few drops of sweet orange, geranium or grapefruit oil.

Childbirth

For labour and birth, clary sage is a powerful oil that helps increase and strengthen labour surges. However, it should NOT be used during pregnancy at is may induce premature labour. It should also NOT be used to kick-start labour as it may cause placenta abruption. Lavender is a wonderful oil to have burning in the background to help keep you and your environment peaceful and calm. Check whether your hospital has a diffuser in the birthing suites; if it doesn't, ask if you can bring your own. If you have a long labour, it may help to mist your face with lavender, neroli or rose oil.

Early motherhood

In the days, weeks and months after bub arrives, it can be hard to find time to nurture yourself. Essential oils are a really easy way to give yourself some love and healing energy. Many citrus oils, such as orange, bergamot, neroli and grapefruit, can help with anxieties and have anti-depressant qualities. Lavender and rose oils also have calming properties. All of these oils are terrific used in diffusers to create a pleasant atmosphere, and bub will love them.

To help your perineum heal after childbirth, you can put witch hazel, lavender and chamomile oil in a warm bath that covers your hips and buttocks, or use them in a spray. This can also help haemorrhoids.

For cracked nipples during breastfeeding, calendula has amazing healing properties. Fennel oil has been known to increase the flow of milk, and eating fennel has the same result.

Note: It is best to avoid using oils directly on your baby without first seeking advice from your care provider or medical doctor.

Sound

Listening to the sounds of nature can be immensely soothing. The sound of rain, running water, waves crashing at the beach, leaves rustling in the wind and the singsong calls of birds all help to create a calm and peaceful atmosphere that induces relaxation. Nature's sounds are generally alluring and peaceful, and can allow deeper, more restful sleep.

You can bring these sounds indoors by listening to nature recordings at work, while cooking dinner or when you're drifting off to sleep. Listening to recordings of nature can be highly beneficial while pregnant and helps you to bond with bub. It's been acknowledged that nature sounds are extremely helpful for soothing newborns and infants. This is especially evident for babies who were exposed to these sounds in utero. You might like to acquire a white noise machine for your child's room, one that includes natural sounds, to help soothe them into sleep.

Taste

An easy way to connect with nature is through eating life-giving and nutrient-filled, plant-based foods. Including foods in your diet that come straight from Mother Nature, such as vegetables, fruits, nuts, seeds and spices, provides a range of healing properties.

That old saying, 'You're eating for two now' happens to be truer than you think. What you eat is being absorbed, processed and passed across the placenta to your baby. Much of the food readily available to us tends to be processed in some way. This includes breakfast cereals, cheese, tinned food, bread, snacks such as crisps, meat products such as bacon, and a lot of the drinks available in supermarkets. While not all processed foods are bad choices (for example, milk needs to be pasteurised to remove harmful bacteria), much of the processed food available has added and/or hidden salt, sugars, fats and preservatives that aren't the best thing for the health of you or your baby.

Where possible, it's best to eat nutrient-rich wholefoods. Examples are: unprocessed grains (for example, brown rice), fruits, vegetables, proteins and dairy products, fresh herbs and spices. A weekly visit to a farmers' market, where wholefoods are more prevalent, will encourage you to stock your fridge and pantry with them. While you can buy wholefoods in supermarkets, it's sometimes too tempting to pick up the highly processed, more convenient foodstuffs that make up the bulk of their product range.

Farmers' markets also tend to sell seasonal foods, which are fresh and, therefore, more nutrient-dense. Alternatively, seasonal boxes delivered to your door each week are available in major cities. These can force you to become quite creative in your cooking, which also stimulates the rich feminine energy that is helpful during the motherhood transition.

Choosing organic food also has health benefits. Organic food is produced without the use of pesticides, synthetic fertilisers, growth hormones and antibiotics, and is not genetically modified. By eating organic food, you aren't ingesting harmful chemicals and passing them across to your baby. It may not be realistic to eat 100% organic, but if you have to limit the organic foods you buy, try to make the best choices. Many authorities suggest that meat and dairy products are the most contaminated foodstuffs and, therefore, should be a priority when buying organic. If you can't buy organic meat, hormone-free is the next best option. A report put out by the Environmental Working Group listed the fruits and vegetables that contain the highest levels of pesticide residues. Helpfully, they also listed the vegetables with the lowest levels.[47]

DIRTY DOZEN+	CLEAN FIFTEEN
Apples	Avocados
Peaches	Avocados
Nectarines	Pineapples
Strawberries	Cabbage
Grapes	Sweet peas (frozen)
Celery	Onions
Spinach	Asparagus
Sweet bell peppers	Mangoes
Cucumbers	Papayas (paw paws)
Cherry tomatoes	Kiwi Fruit
Snap peas	Eggplant
Potatoes	Grapefruit
Hot pepper	Rockmelon
Kale / collard greens	Cauliflower
	Sweet potatoes

This information is provided so you can make informed decisions, but don't think that the foods listed in the 'dirty dozen+' should be avoided altogether; it's always better to eat fresh wholefoods than not eat them.

Drinking lots of water also has tremendous health benefits for pregnancy, birth and early motherhood. Water helps your body absorb essential nutrients and transport vitamins, minerals and hormones across the placenta. Not only does it hydrate your growing body, it also increases the volume of amniotic fluid that surrounds your baby and flushes toxins out of your system. Keeping well hydrated during labour and birth is also very helpful. Drinking around twelve glasses of water a day is recommended during pregnancy, and you should increase that by an extra glass or two while breastfeeding.

In our family, we link our food with nature by saying a short blessing to the earth and Mother Nature before we eat:

'We give thanks to the earth that provided this food and the hands that prepared it. May it nourish our mind, body and spirit so we can do amazing things.'

EXERCISE

1) Take the 'Seven-Day Grounding Challenge'. For five minutes a day for seven days, find a patch of grass, kick off your shoes and connect with the earth.

2) At least once a month, find a natural body of water—the ocean, a waterfall or a natural spring—and ground your energy by spending some time there.

3) At least once a week, take a bath or swim in a pool to relieve pressure on your growing and expanding body.

4) Find a patch of nature and observe how each of your senses engages with nature.
   - What do you see?
   - What do you hear?
   - What do you smell?
   - What can you touch with your hands and feet?

   Observe how you feel when you connect with each of your senses.

5) Keep note of what you are eating, and see if you can find ways to increase your intake of nutrient-rich wholefoods, organic where possible.

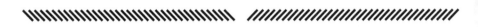

COMING HOME NATURALLY

While it's easy enough to find ways to connect with nature, even for urban dwellers, there's no reason why you shouldn't also find a way to make your home environment more natural.

Your home is your sanctuary and will likely be the place where you'll spend most of your time when bub arrives. It's worth spending time now to create a positive environment at home and eliminate toxins so they aren't passed across to your developing baby.

There are many ways to go about this and, depending on your current lifestyle, it may take a while to phase all of these options into your life. That's okay, as even small changes will have a positive influence on your baby.

Detox your home

We live in a society obsessed with germs. It alarms me how often advertising sends messages that show happy families that are germ-free but surrounded by chemicals. When I looked into many of these products, they contain harmful substances best kept out of the reach of children. But what about their use during pregnancy?

The chemicals you use to clean and kill germs and insects are also entering your lungs when you breathe and potentially being absorbed through your skin. Those same chemicals are likely to be passed to your baby. I know you're motivated to give your baby the best start in life, so without sounding like a preacher on a soap box, it's a good idea to look out for natural alternatives.

Supermarkets stock high-quality cleaning products that are earth-friendly and toxin-free. However, you can easily make cleaning products yourself with lemon, baking soda and vinegar, which are fabulous cleaners and kill ninety-nine per cent of germs. Microfibre cleaning products are another excellent alternative.

It should also be noted that allowing your baby to be exposed to some level of germs can be good for their immune system—a mounting body of research suggests that exposing infants to germs may offer them greater protection from illnesses such as allergies and asthma later in life. You'll find that when baby is old enough, they'll pop everything in their mouth—this is probably nature's way of exposing them to microorganisms that are good for them, as well as offering them protection from illnesses later in life. So don't fret if you don't have the time or energy to clean your house regularly when you have a newborn.

A la naturale cleaning product recipe

Ingredients

500ml vinegar

500ml water

1 spoonful baking soda

A few drops of dishwashing detergent

A few drops of tea tree oil or lemon oil

Method

Mix together ingredients (the baking soda will make it bubble a bit, but don't worry about that). Pour into old bottles to store, and put some in a spray bottle for all-purpose use on bench tops, etc. Use undiluted.

As the ingredients are all natural they can be used on most surfaces, including the bathroom. For heavy-duty cleaning you can mix together a little vinegar with a generous amount of baking soda to make a scrub.

Detox your body

Once you've got your environment back into a more natural state, you can turn your attention to your body.

Did you know that sixty per cent of what you put on your body is absorbed through your skin and into your bloodstream? This is true for whatever you're using to wash, cleanse, moisturise, shampoo, condition and perfume your body. Conventional skin-care products that you buy in supermarkets or chemists are chock-full of parabens, chemicals and sulphates. Parabens are preservatives that have been linked to breast cancer through their ability to mimic oestrogen. Sulphates are effective cleansing and foaming agents that can have a degenerative effect on cell membranes. Unfortunately, some of these agents are entering your bloodstream and, ultimately, being passed to your baby.

The great news is that it's quite easy to find natural, toxin-free and affordable skincare products, including body washes, shampoos, conditioners, and make-up. Major supermarkets are now stocking toxin-free products and you can find a wide range in health food stores.

DID YOU KNOW?

There are a number of common nasties in body-care products that are best avoided.

INGREDIENTS	REASON TO AVOID
Butylated hydroxyanisole (BHA) and butylated hydroxytoluene (BHT)	Endocrine disruptors and suspected carcinogenic.
Diethanolamine (DEA), monsethasolamine (MEA) and triethanolamine (TEA)	Skin irritant, causes contact dermatitis, suspected carginogen.
Parabens (Methyl, butyl, ethyl, propyl)	Endocrine disruptor (mimics estrogen).
Parfum/ synthetic fragrance	Often undisclosed ingredients and can trigger allergies, asthma, cancer and neurotoxicity.

Polyethylene glycol (PEG)	Can be contaminated with 1,4-dioxane, a known carginogen.
Sodium lauryl sulphate (SLS) and sodium laureth sulphate (SLES)	Can be contaminated with 1,4-dioxane, a known carginogen.
Triclosan	Endocrine disruptor and suspected carcinogen.
Methylisothiazolinone (MI)	Used in babywipes and wide range of body-care products. Can cause contact dermatitis.

When detoxing your body, it's also important to consider the bottles and containers we use to store our food and drinks. I'm sure you're aware of BPA, otherwise known as bisphenol A, and you may have noticed how many storage containers now advertise being BPA-free. However, not many of us are aware of the impacts BPA has on our bodies, especially for a foetus in the womb. BPA is an endocrine disruptor, which means that it interferes with the body's endocrine system and has adverse effects on the developmental, reproductive, neurological and immune systems. Research shows that endocrine disruptors may pose the greatest risk during prenatal and early postnatal development, when organ and neural systems are forming.[48]

BPA mimics naturally occurring hormones in the body, such as oestrogen, which means the body doesn't stop it from crossing the placenta. Therefore, it's of utmost importance to avoid as much BPA as possible during pregnancy and post-partum. Thankfully, it's easy to find BPA-free containers and drink bottles, but bear in mind that plastic replacements are also likely to be endocrine disruptors, so opt for glass or aluminium. There are also some sources of BPA that you may not be aware of, including:

- The lining of food tins.
- Plastic, such as soft drink bottles, water bottles, disposable coffee cup lids, plastic toys.
- Receipts printed on thermal paper (unless you need a receipt, say no when it's offered).
- The inside of lids on glass bottles.

This information isn't meant to instil fear; it's about providing knowledge and raising awareness. It's probably impossible to fully avoid BPA and other endocrine disruptors, but it's possible to take steps to minimise exposure.

Connecting with nature is the final point on the connection compass, but that doesn't mean it's the end of your journey. There is no beginning or end to a compass. If you stand at its centre, you will see that it is essentially a circle. And from its centre, in the eye of the storm of your motherhood journey, the compass will help point you in the right direction—towards connecting with yourself, with your baby, with your partner and community, and with Mother Nature herself. The work you have done up to now is a wonderful start, but you will be a mother for the rest of your life, and it is just as important to work at maintaining your connections as it was to forge them. The final chapter will help you do that.

PART 6:

MAINTAINING CONNECTIONS

'Every time you praise something, every time you appreciate something, every time you feel good about something, you're telling the Universe, "More of this, please. More of this, please."'

ABRAHAM

The main thrust of this book has been about understanding the connection compass, which helps you navigate your journey to motherhood by exploring four distinct but key themes.

This section helps bring those four points together, with a range of simple daily activities that help maintain those connections. It's like running a marathon—you learn about the different pillars involved— such as training programmes, nutrition and equipment that can help you achieve your goal—but unless you wake up each day and consistently get out of bed and go for a run, it will be an uphill battle to actually last the distance and cross the finish line.

None of the techniques listed here are rocket science or particularly ground-breaking. They are, however, simple, tried-and-tested techniques that help people get into a more positive frame of mind. They're known to help raise energy. They help people change neural pathways to create more palatable behaviours and beliefs. When people use these techniques, they feel good.

That's what maintaining connections boils down to: Finding ways to make you, your baby and the people around you feel good and full of joy. It's really as simple as that.

Use these techniques like a menu. Pick and choose the activities that resonate with you. There is no right or wrong selection here. These techniques have been chosen because they don't take up a lot of time, which is important because you're a busy professional baking a baby and soon you'll have your hands very full. These activities are specifically designed to be short, sharp and effective.

AFFIRMATIONS

Time required: One to ten minutes

Frequency: Several times daily

Recommended for: Anxiety management, positive mindset, personal growth

In very simple terms, an affirmation is a positive statement that describes a specific situation that you would like to be visible in your life. It is a statement about who you are and what you can become.

Most of us are familiar with the voice in our head that's all too ready to squash our ideas and hopes and remind us of our fears and inadequacies. It's the voice of the subconscious and it's hardwired through years of habit to focus on negative and destructive thoughts and beliefs. Your subconscious mind accepts negative thoughts and beliefs just as easily, if not more readily, than positive ones.

But we can adopt new thought patterns by training our brain to overcome negative thoughts, ultimately re-wiring neural pathways and changing existing beliefs. Saying affirmations regularly, with conviction and passion, is one way of doing this.

Consciously, deliberately and consistently reciting affirmations will hardwire a new circuit in your brain. Eventually, the positive belief will represent the path of least resistance for your lazy brain. Your positive belief will be the first thought that pops up in a difficult situation, and gradually your negative and limiting thought is pushed from your mind. The positive thought will become the default.

Regular use of affirmations embeds your new beliefs, which, in turn, allows you to respond more calmly and with greater control to the challenges that present themselves in your parenting journey. This presents you with an attitude of capability that means you can say 'I've got this' when you hit a stumbling block.

And believe me, when you enter your parenting journey there won't be any shortage of stumbling blocks. Through your pregnancy, childbirth and then as your baby grows and develops you'll keep hitting more stumbling blocks and finding more things to learn about. It's a never-ending learning process.

After you make daily affirmations a habit, you'll feel something shift. You'll find that you respond in a calmer manner to the day-to-day challenges and, in turn, your baby will be calmer as they respond to your energy.

Creating affirmations

There is a bit of an art to affirmations; using the following tips will help them penetrate your neural pathways more easily:

- Make yourself the central actor: When you use the words 'I, my, me', you're making a powerful statement about your identity and intentions. The result? Your subconscious mind pays attention. For example, '*I* have what it takes to be a great parent'.
- Use affirmations in the present tense: When you do this, you're declaring that it's already happening. This helps you believe that the statement is true right now. To use the above example, 'I *have* what it takes to be a great parent'.
- Use positive and direct language: Avoid using double negatives and words that have a negative connotation. For example, 'no debt' is better described as 'financial freedom'.
- Word the affirmations as if you have already achieved the result, not as if you're moving towards it. For example, 'I am confident in my decisions as a mother', even if you may not feel that way now.

Using affirmations:

- Use affirmations multiple times a day.
- Say your affirmations out loud.
- Use language that is meaningful to you.
- Say your affirmations to yourself in the mirror.

- Record your affirmations on your phone and play them back to yourself.
- Sing and dance your affirmations.

\\\\\\\\\\\\\\\\\\\\\\\\\\\\ **EXERCISE** /////////////////////////

1) Go back to the Connect with you section and revisit the intentions and the fears, expectations and blockages that you uncovered about your pregnancy, birth and when bub arrives.

2) Look at the wording you used for each of your intentions and, if they aren't already in the present tense, with you as the central actor, reword them so they meet the formula above.

3) Now look at your expectations and fears. Can you turn them from negative assertions into a series of positive statements that follow the same formula?

Here are some examples:
- 'I'm terrified of giving birth' can become 'I'm confident to give birth to my baby'.
- 'I'm worried I'll lose who I am when I don't to go work every day and stay at home with a baby' can turn into 'Becoming a mother provides further depth to my identity'.
- 'I'm afraid a careless move will result in my baby being dropped or hurt' can become 'I am confident and adept in handling my baby'.
- 'I don't know what to do with my baby' can become 'I trust my parenting instincts', 'My baby constantly teaches me' or 'Support comes to me when I need it'.

- 'Will I have enough money when I have a baby?' can become 'I'm grateful for the abundance that flows into our lives to meet all our needs'.

4) Once you have your list of affirmations, tap into your creativity to design them, record them and plaster them around the house where you will see them often.

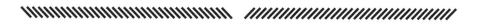

You can find affirmations that suit pregnancy, birth and early motherhood on my website: www.theconnectedmama.com.

BREATHING EXERCISES

Time required: Five minutes

Recommended frequency: As required

Recommended for: Relaxation, stress management, pain management, re-energising

Breathing exercises are one of the easiest and simplest ways to transform your mood. Once you get into the rhythm of breathing exercises, you can transform how you feel and control your nervous system in a matter of seconds. Extensive research has proven that rhythmic breathing causes complex, beneficial physiological changes, including an improved supply of oxygen to the blood, more efficient brain functioning and better disposal of bodily wastes.[49] The benefits are quite astounding. You can boost your energy, deepen your relaxation and enhance your inner concentration.

If you pay attention to your breathing, you'll find that shallow and rapid breathing is a classic response to stress. Yet, with deep breathing, you can control your nervous system and encourage your body to relax. This is a helpful tool for pregnancy, birth and when you are feeling stressed or anxious in the early days with bub and want to calm down your emotions.

Breathing exercises are free and are something you can do at any time of the day, in any place and without any external resource. There are many types of breathing exercises, so you're bound to find something that works well for you.

Many breathing exercises involve counting, which helps your mind to focus and quiets busy thoughts. For example, you can count up to a chosen number, such as four, six or eight, while inhaling, then exhale for the same count. I find counting while breathing is a great way to mindfully focus attention so I don't drift away with my thoughts. However, once you are breathing in a rhythm you can drop the counting and just inhale and exhale naturally.

Relaxation breathing

Relaxation breathing is a simple breathing mantra that I discovered in hypnobirthing preparation and still use to drop into a deep state of relaxation. It has a number of applications. It can be used during labour for maintaining relaxation between contractions. It's also a wonderful exercise to use during pregnancy and after your baby is born if you're feeling stressed or anxious and need to calm down quickly. It's a fuss-free, quick way to top up your energy so you have more resilience and patience to get you through whatever difficulty you're facing.

It's a simple technique: Breathe in to the count of four. Breathe out to the count of eight.

You can use this mantra:

In...two...three...four...Out...two...three...four...five...six...seven... eight...

Repeat three times at first, then gradually increase to several minutes at a time.

If you practice this breathing mantra on a regular basis—say when you wake up and before you go to bed, or when you're stopped at the traffic lights—it can become an anchor. This means you can trigger a sense of calm right from the first breath, which makes it a valuable everyday tool.

'Some more' breathing

I often use this technique during meditation as a way to direct my attention away from my thoughts. This exercise is suited more for early motherhood, after you've given birth. The exercise involves holding your breath for a number of counts, so I recommend you check with your care provider before doing this activity during pregnancy.

Deeply inhale through your nose until your lungs are full, counting slowly. You may get up to a count of four or six. Once your lungs are full, hold for up to a count of four, then breathe in some more until your lungs are at full capacity. Hold for another couple of counts and then exhale slowly through your nose for the same count or a little longer, forcing your breath out from the back of your throat.

ENERGY BALANCING

Time required: Five minutes

Frequency: As required

Recommended for: Altering energy balance

Our bodies have two meridians of energy—masculine and feminine. The left side is feminine and the right side is masculine. According to ancient Swara Yogic teachings, we regulate our energy and nervous systems by alternating the nostril we breathe through. In the mid-1890s, this was described by German physician Richard Kayser as the nasal cycle, indicating alternating partial congestion and decongestion of the nasal cavities. While we may think we breathe through both nostrils, most of us are actually only breathing through a single nostril and the other nostril partially congests to restrict airflow.

When you're breathing through your right nostril, you're activating your masculine energy, which can give you more physical energy. It also activates the left hemisphere of your brain (the logical side) and makes it dominant. The opposite happens when you're breathing through your left nostril; you engage your feminine energy and relax and calm your physical energy. It also activates the right hemisphere (the creative side) of your brain.[50]

A natural nasal cycle would see us alternate nostrils regularly and for equal intervals. However, for most of us it's out of balance. There are some different exercises you can practise to regulate these energies and allow you to become centred or activate a particular energy as needed.

To centre the two energies

Alternate nostril breathing gradually cleanses and aligns your masculine and feminine energy into a position of harmony. The following exercise can be used both during pregnancy and when bub arrives. If you're pregnant, I recommend that you skip the steps of holding your breath and introduce them after you have your baby.

Deeply inhale through the left nostril for a count of four, closing the right nostril with your thumb. Hold your breath, closing both nostrils for a count of four if you can manage it. Exhale through the right nostril to the count of eight, keeping your left nostril closed with your index finger. Now, inhale through your right nostril, keeping your left nostril closed. Hold your breath, closing both nostrils, to the count of four. Exhale through your left nostril, keeping your right nostril closed, to the count of eight. You can repeat this slowly and rhythmically for a number of minutes.

If you're pregnant, just breathe in and out without holding your breath. After bub arrives, you can gradually increase the amount of time you hold your breath as your practice progresses. Increasing the count by multiples of four works well. Begin with 4:4:8 (i.e., breathe in for four counts, hold for four counts and exhale for four counts), then extend to 4:8:8, and then to 4:16:8.

To engage a particular energy

As professional women are often operating in the dominant masculine energy, it is useful to have a breathing exercise that will help you to engage with the feminine. To increase your feminine energy, sit quietly and close your right nostril with your right thumb. Breathe deeply and slowly, inhaling and exhaling through your left nostril for three minutes at a time.

There may be times when you want to engage your masculine energy. For example, when your baby arrives and you want an energy boost. When you need more masculine energy, do the opposite breathing technique. Close your left nostril with your left thumb, and breathe deeply and slowly through your right nostril for three minutes at a time.

FEAR RELEASE

Time required: Fifteen seconds

Frequency: As required

Recommended for: Releasing fears

In addition to the fear-release exercise in the *Connect with You* section, you may find it useful to recite the 'Litany Against Fear' featured in Frank Herbert's novel *Dune*. The novel features a group of powerful women—the Bene Gesserit—who take their bodies and minds through years of physical and mental conditioning to obtain superhuman powers and abilities. They use the 'Litany Against Fear' to focus their minds and calm themselves in times of peril. During your transition to motherhood, you may find you need to be superhuman sometimes, and the words of the litany may resonate with you.

While the breathing exercises in *Connect with You* were designed to be completed in a structured way to achieve long-term effects, you can recite the litany as a quick-fix when unforeseen fears get in the way of your daily functioning. Simply reciting the following words in your head can help you move through a difficult moment, as it allows you to acknowledge and feel the fear, without getting caught up in it.

I must not fear.
Fear is the mind-killer.
Fear is the little-death that brings total obliteration.
I will face my fear.

I will permit it to pass over me and through me.
And when it has gone past I will turn the inner eye to see its path.
Where the fear has gone there will be nothing.
Only I will remain.

GRATITUDE

Time required: Five minutes
Frequency: Daily
Recommended for: Emotional health, positive mindset, raising your energy vibration

It has been said that feeling appreciation is the closest we can come to experiencing godliness. I'm not sure about that, but I know that being grateful—and looking for things to be grateful for—feels pretty darn good.

Digging a bit deeper, it's not surprising that it's completely backed up by science. Studies by Robert Emmons, the world's leading scientific expert on gratitude, show that keeping a gratitude journal or reflecting on things you feel grateful for has physical, psychological and social benefits, ultimately leading to an increase in happiness and a decrease in the incidence of negative states.[51]

According to Phil Watkins, psychologist and author of the book *Gratitude and the Good Life*, being in a gratitude mind frame sets off what is called a positivity bias.[52] This means that you tend to pay attention to positive things in your life instead of focusing on negative events. As you direct your attention to positive elements, you attract happiness and positivity in even greater measure. Therefore, gratitude is an amplifier of the good in your life.

You receive what you give. So if you give gratitude on a daily basis, you will receive a lot more to be grateful for.

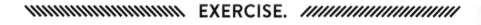 **EXERCISE.**

Keep a daily gratitude diary.

1) In your trusty journal (or you may wish to buy a beautiful journal dedicated to this process), write down three to five things that happened during the day that you're grateful for.

2) If possible, do this before going to bed, so that you drift off to sleep with an energy of appreciation.

3) Try to keep this diary for at least three weeks. With repetition comes habit.

If you find that it's difficult to write down the points you're grateful for, say them out loud to your baby. Whether your baby is in utero or in your arms, this is a wonderful habit to start with them. Juan, now almost three, understands gratitude and each night rattles off the things that he is grateful for.

\\ ///////////////////////////////////////

Keeping a gratitude diary can be challenging at first, but soon it becomes a fabulous exercise in looking out for things to appreciate. Here are some tips for your gratitude points:

- Be as specific as possible.
- You can be grateful for people, things and events.
- It's okay to be grateful for negative outcomes that you were able to avoid, prevent or turn into something positive.
- We adapt to positive events and may become numb if we repeat the same points too often, so try to be grateful for something different each day. This will get you into the habit of looking out for and remembering positive things in your life.

As an example, here are five things I'm grateful for today:

1. I am grateful that Leland cooked dinner as it gave me a chance to be organised and fold Juan's cloth nappies.
2. I am grateful that I finally met Lucinda's mother at day care today.
3. I am grateful that the barista accidentally upsized my flat white from regular to large this morning.
4. I am grateful that Leland put Juan to bed tonight so I could concentrate on writing this chapter.
5. I am grateful that I was able to have a good belly laugh while watching a silly YouTube video.

LAUGHTER

Time required: Thirty seconds plus

Frequency: Daily

Recommended for: General well-being, stress management, positive mindset

I'm sure you've heard the saying, 'Laughter is the best medicine.' There is certainly an element of truth to that saying.

Laughter is known to mitigate the effects of stress, by reducing stress-making hormones in the body, such as cortisol and adrenaline. At the same time, it increases dopamine and serotonin activity and triggers endorphins, which enhances your feelings of health and wellbeing.

But I don't need to tell you that, right? You know that laughter feels good.

Make time in your day for laughter. You know what sort of humour you have, so perhaps search for clips on YouTube that appeal to this sense of humour, watch some feel good comedy shows and movies, subscribe to blogs and pages that give you some giggles. You might have some great friends who make you laugh. You may even want to take it a step further and sign up to a Laughter Yoga class. You might feel a bit silly at first, but laughter is tremendously healing, as it releases your stored energy and emotions.

\\\\\\\\\\\\\\\\\\\\\\\\\\\\\\\ **EXERCISE** ///////////////////////

- Take out your trusty journal and write down 3 things or people who make you laugh.
- See if you can build in activities into your day that allows you to tap into the good feelings you get from those things or people.
- To go one step further, keep note of when and how long you laugh for each day, and see if you can build upon that each day.

\\ ///////////////////////////////

MEDITATION

Time required: Thirty seconds plus

Frequency: Daily

Recommended for: General well-being, stress management, anxiety management, positive mindset, raising your energy vibration.

Many of us are aware of the benefits of meditation, such as better focus, reduced anxiety and less stress. It allows us, for a few minutes, to stop engaging in the busy-ness of our minds and allow ourselves to 'be'. It brings us back into our bodies and recalibrates our system.

Meditation is a truly exquisite practice for pregnancy, birth and after your baby comes. It provides space for us to reset and welcome peace and allowance into our lives and the lives of our baby and family.

In prioritising our day, it should be very high on our list—as important as eating breakfast or lunch. Yet, how many of us actually find time to meditate or even know how to?

Understanding meditation

I believe there are a lot of misconceptions around meditation. For example, that to get the benefits you need to spend a long time meditating, that you need to go to a class to learn, that you have to be sitting cross-legged on the floor, that you have to empty your mind.

Don't let these misconceptions put you off. You can meditate for any length of time—even thirty seconds or a minute will have benefits. You don't need to attend a class to learn how to meditate. You don't need to be sitting cross-legged on the floor. You can meditate anywhere—on the bus, as you're walking down the street, when you're cleaning, cooking, showering, at your desk in the office. You certainly don't need to empty your mind—that is probably the main reason a lot of people give up.

There are many different ways to meditate, but the one that seems to resonate well with most people is mindfulness meditation. This is where you focus on a specific thing, such as:

- Your breathing;
- A sensation in your body; or
- Something in your environment—the birds singing outside, the traffic passing by, or the fans spinning in the room.

You can also follow guided meditation scripts if that helps you focus and visualise. You can find scripts for every circumstance in your life, and I have created and shared a few that resonate for pregnancy and the transition to motherhood.

Other meditation techniques involve following a mantra. The reason they work so well is because they allow you to fall into a rhythm and your attention is directed to the chant, which means that busy thoughts are kept at bay.

Meditation can be a personal practice and the key to success is finding something that suits you. You'll know when it suits you—it will feel right and feel good.

If you aren't accustomed to meditating, it's worth noting that meditation is not something to force—in fact, it can't be forced. Think of meditation as a chance to relax. If your attention wanders, that's fine; simply acknowledge it and direct your attention back to what you were doing. That's why the use of scripts or anchors such as focusing on your breathing and observing the noises around you are widely used in meditation. They bring you back when your thoughts start to wander.

It's impossible to still your thoughts; the key to meditation is to not get caught up in them.

You might find that during meditation some fabulous ideas and solutions to problems arise. These can be a terrific by-product of meditation and you don't necessarily want to suppress those thoughts.

I get a lot of ideas and answers during meditation and I often park them in my mind to write down afterwards. If my mind starts to get caught up in the details of the idea, it's best that I get out of meditation, write down the idea for further consideration later and return to a meditative state.

Putting meditation into practice

In this wonderful time of transformation in your life, you can use meditation for different purposes. You can use it to relax and find some peace to centre yourself and your energies. This is very beneficial for keeping daily stresses at bay and keeping a calm and even temperament for baby. Otherwise, you can use meditation to connect with your baby—as a chance to bond.

The following exercises provide a combination of those two approaches.

Mindfulness

Mindfulness is about being present and aware in the activity you're doing. Jon Kabat-Zinn, a leading global authority on the use of mindfulness, defines it as 'paying attention in a particular way: on purpose, in the present moment and non-judgementally.'

For example, if you're washing your hair, you would feel the water as it flows onto your head and body, you would raise your face to meet the stream of water and feel the pressure of the water, take note of the water temperature. You would feel the sensation as you pour the shampoo into the palm of your hand. You would feel how the texture changes when you lather it into your hair, feel your fingers as they massage your scalp. You would notice how your scalp feels as you wash the shampoo out of your hair.

This is one example, and you can also use this technique when cooking, cleaning, breastfeeding your baby or in any number of other daily scenarios. Just spend a few minutes really observing what is happening and the sensations you feel in your body. An important part of mindfulness is non-judgement. Instead of identifying particular thoughts, observations and sensations as good or bad, right or wrong, just acknowledge them for what they are, with openness and awareness.

Mindfulness example in practice

A few days ago I found myself in a wonderful meditation on the bus. I closed my eyes and let myself sway in tune with the movements of the bus. I felt the warmth of the sun flickering through the trees and roofs onto my face. I listened to the bus accelerate and brake, noticing the hydraulics as the driver opened the door to let more passengers on. I observed the smell of the perfume of the lady in front of me and the sweat and stale cigarette smoke lingering on the jacket of the young man standing next to me. I listened to the silence of the early morning passengers. I focused on the distant sounds of someone listening to music through their earphones. All of this happened in mere minutes, no one on the bus was any the wiser, but it was enough to immerse myself in a deep mindful meditation, becoming recharged and ready to start the day on the right note.

Heart connection meditation with baby during pregnancy

This is a wonderful meditation to practice while you're pregnant.

Find a peaceful environment where you feel safe and comfortable.

Slowly inhale and, as you do so, welcome love into your being.

As you exhale, imagine sending that love from your heart down to your baby.

Inhale again, bringing more love into your lungs and down to your heart.

Exhale and send more love from your heart to your baby.

Imagine your baby becoming more and more relaxed as she feels more welcome in your life with each new breath.

Observe and feel her movements as you send her love.

Now, as you inhale, feel your baby's love rise up to meet the love you are sending her.

Feel both of your love connect, grow and expand.

Feel your combined love radiate through your body.

Feel it flow from your womb up to your heart, into your shoulders and down your arms, through to your fingertips.

Feel the love flow up your neck to your chin; feel your jaw open and relax.

Feel your cheeks relax, your eyes relax, your brow and forehead relax. Feel the top of your head relax as your and your baby's love flows right through your entire being.

Now feel love flow down your legs, through your feet and into your toes.

Feel the love extend into the earth below you, forming roots and a connection deep into the earth.

Feel the support and nourishment the earth provides back into you, flowing into your base, providing you with the strength and fortitude you require for your motherhood journey.

You are connected, with your baby and with the earth.

You are nourished, nurtured, supported and protected. So is your baby.

You are both a complete expression of love.

Deeply inhale and appreciate the love that's flowing through your being, the love which you share with your baby.

Slowly exhale and bring your attention back to the room.

Place your hands on your pregnant belly and say a word of thanks to the peace now flowing within you and through your baby.

Heart connection meditation with baby

This exercise is a lovely way to form a connection with your baby and also be supported yourself by sacred feminine energy. Do this activity when feeding your baby, holding them close to your heart.

Find a place where you and your baby will be comfortable and supported; this may be on the sofa or in bed propped up by pillows. Sit in a restful position and invite your baby to join you in the meditation.

Breathe in deeply and concentrate on your lungs filling up with life-giving air. Exhale slowly.

Breathe in deeply again, feeling the sensation of air entering and exiting your nostrils, your throat, your lungs, as you inhale and exhale.

Repeat this breath rhythm again, over and over until you feel a sense of relaxation overcome you.

Now bring your attention to the top of your head. Feel your scalp, forehead, cheeks and jaw relax.

Relax your neck, your shoulders, your arms, your hands and your fingers.

Relax your chest, your abdomen, your hips, your legs, your knees, your ankles and your toes.

Invite your baby to also relax their features.

Now you are fully relaxed, feel your baby's body against your warm body.

Feel your heart beat in time with your baby's tiny heartbeat. Both of your hearts communicate love, trust, compassion and protection in each beat.

Imagine an invisible string drawn between your heart and your baby's heart. Imagine a light pulsating back and forth along the string between your hearts with each heartbeat.

Now imagine this white light turning pink. A rush of love travels back and forth between you. Pure, clean love, pulsating with each heartbeat and each breath.

As you take in your next breath you see the light grow a stronger shade of pink as more love flows between you and your baby.

The light starts to pulsate from both of your hearts and starts flowing up your bodies to the tip of your heads and down to the bottom of your toes.

You imagine yourself and your baby glowing in the pink light of love.

The light spreads to the room around you, cleansing the air and creating an atmosphere filled with love.

Now, as you take your next breath, be aware of the air passing through your nostrils, down your throat, into your lungs. The light between you and your baby turns white.

This time it radiates a sense of peace and confidence. A deep sense of knowing that no matter what you face in the day ahead, the two of you have a connection that will rise above all else.

You feel a sense of relief.

As you deeply breathe in once more, place your hand on your baby's forehead and send them a blessing of peace and love.

As you inhale again, silently thank your baby for your beautiful heart-to-heart connection and give them a gentle kiss as you slowly exhale.

Take in one final deep breath and smile as you exhale, giving thanks.

Five-minute meditation for centering

This exercise will help you to become more present in the here and now when your thoughts and emotions are particularly scattered.

Give yourself permission, when you take your next breath, to be more conscious.

Allow your breath to bring you into the present, to the here and now.

Gently let go of the past and worries of the future.

Just allow yourself to be present in this moment.

Feel the hard floor beneath your feet, supporting you.

Feel the air against your skin, enveloping your body.

Breathe deeply in through your nose.

As you inhale, feel your lungs expand like an inflating balloon.

As you exhale, expel any tension and negative emotion.

Relax your shoulders down like ice melting on a hot day.

Relax your jaw, allow your tongue to rest gently between your teeth.

Notice your breath and allow it to bring you into the present moment.
Quiet your mind.
Picture a stream in front of you, its water gently flowing.
When thoughts enter your awareness, place them in this stream and watch them float away.
Bring your attention back to your breath.
As you inhale, feel your lungs expand like an inflating balloon.
As you exhale, expel any tension and negative emotion.
Enjoy being in the present moment.
Begin to nurture an inner peace.
A silence within, filled with love.
Slowly breathe in and slowly exhale. Repeat this pattern for as long as you wish.
When you're ready, bring your attention back to the room.
Say a word of thanks to the peace now flowing within you.

Audio versions for each of the above meditations are available for download on my website: www.theconnectedmama.com.

ME-TIME

Time required: Ten minutes

Frequency: Three times per week

Recommended for: Emotional health, stress management

As a mother you are at the very foundation of your family's well-being. Therefore, it's vital that you nourish yourself and take time out to look after yourself so you can, in turn, nourish your family.

'Me-time' is time taken to slow down and be comfortable in your own company. It's a great chance to relax and provides some space for you to connect inwardly with yourself. Taking time out for yourself is a nurturing and beautiful habit to start during pregnancy, as you give yourself permission to slow down and truly appreciate you, and the miracle that is unfolding in your body.

When it comes to motherhood, however, taking time out for yourself is a crucial action you can take for your emotional and mental health. While in the early days it may seem a luxury or even impossible, getting some 'me-time' is the single greatest thing that I hear mothers say they miss.

When you become a mother, especially if you're the main caregiver, it can be hard to let go of your baby and entrust them to the care of someone else, even their father. But as hard as this is, it's so important for your emotional health and your sanity.

I remember a time when my son was a few weeks old and I needed to run an errand. I lived in one of Brisbane's trendier suburbs and was only a short walk from the shops and cafes. I felt unimaginable freedom at being able to walk by myself up to the shops. Even though I don't think I had showered yet that day and was wearing a shirt completely covered in Juan's milk spew, I felt like a million dollars. It was such a simple thing, but I can still remember the feeling two years later.

Another very fond memory is the first time I rode my bicycle after Juan's birth. Juan was several months old by then. I remember flying along the Brisbane River at great speed, feeling the wind in my hair (well, I was wearing a helmet, but I thought I could feel the wind in my hair). It lifted my soul even though it was only a half-hour ride.

Taking me-time doesn't have to take a lot of time, and you'll soon find out how long you can be away from your baby before missing them starts to spoil your me-time experience. You may very well be able to thoroughly enjoy a night out with the girls, but in my experience I really missed Juan after forty-five minutes; after I crossed that threshold I didn't enjoy myself anymore. I found that short bursts of ten minutes were advantageous and realistic. The important thing is to find out what works for you and your circumstances and, most importantly, fills your being with joy.

Taking me-time also doesn't need to involve someone else stepping in to look after your child. You might find that by rearranging your priorities, as discussed in *Connect with you*, you're able to fit in thirty minutes of yoga, watch your favourite show on Netflix, create a quick sketch or piece of artwork, catch up with an old friend on the phone, bake a cake, or do whatever you can that makes you feel great and doesn't involve leaving the house.

EXERCISE

- Proactively organise a date for yourself at least three times a week, even if it's just a ten-minute walk around the block.
- In your trusty journal, write down what you did during your 'me-time' date and how it made you feel. This way you can have a ready reference of the activities that work for you when you need a boost.

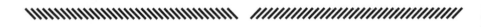

PRANA CLEANSING

Time required: Five minutes
Frequency: Daily if possible
Recommended for: Starting the day, re-energising, stress management

Prana is a Sanskrit word that means life-force or the vital energy that flows through all things in the universe.[53] This exercise is a great activity to start the day, or to settle into the evening after a long day as the movement addresses physical and emotional imbalances.

This prana cleansing exercise engages both feminine and masculine energies. As the movements activate both sides of the body, often in symmetrical movements, it allows for centred energy and balance.

The following exercise was shown to me in a meditation class and was adapted from Master Choa Kok Sui's teachings. If you do this exercise while pregnant, ensure you have a wall or some furniture close-by to help you keep your balance, and keep the movements slow.

- Stand up straight, feet shoulder-width apart, with knees slightly bent.
- Lift your right leg and circle your ankle twelve times clockwise, then twelve times anti-clockwise. Repeat with your left ankle.
- Place your knees together, bend down and grip your knees with your hands (if you can). Circle your knees twelve times clockwise and then twelve times anti-clockwise.
- Hold onto the wall or a piece of furniture, then lift your right leg out to your side, keeping it straight, and circle it twelve times clockwise and then twelve times anti-clockwise. Repeat for your left leg.
- Stand up straight, bend your knees slightly, place your hands on your hips and circle your pelvis twelve times clockwise and then twelve times anti-clockwise.
- Stand up straight, bend your knees slightly with your feet shoulder-width apart, and extend your arms out straight to each side. Twist your body from your waist so your left arm is behind your back and your right arm is outstretched in front of your body. Then twist back to the centre, swapping your arms to the opposite position. Repeat this twenty-four times.
- Still standing straight, knees bent and feet shoulder-width apart, lift your right arm and rotate it from the shoulder in twelve clockwise circular movements. It's the same movement as freestyle swimming, but with the arm quite straight. Then move your arm backwards in an anti-clockwise movement twelve times, as if you were doing backstroke. Repeat for the left arm.
- The next movements must be done carefully as they involve the delicate muscles in your neck. Slowly and carefully move your head to the right at a ninety-degree angle and bring back to the centre looking ahead. Then slowly move your head to the left at a ninety-degree angle and then to the centre again. Repeat this slowly twelve times on each side.

- Lastly, carefully and slowly lift your head up so you're looking at the ceiling and then tuck your chin into your neck and look down to your belly. If you're doing this while pregnant, say hello and send some love to your baby every time you look down. Repeat this twelve times.
- Finish the exercise by gently shaking off your body.
- You can find a video of this activity on my website: www. theconnectedmama.com.

VISUALISATION

Time required: Ten minutes

Frequency: Twice a week

Recommended for: Times of doubt or uncertainty, regular reinforcement of your intentions, positive mindset

Back in the *Connect with you* section, you set intentions for how you wanted your pregnancy, birth and early motherhood to be. To help you stay on path with those intentions, visualisation is a powerful tool that is proven to work.

Top athletes use it. Top business people use it. Visualisation affects many cognitive processes, such as motor control, attention, perception and memory, and prepares your brain for the actual events. Your subconscious can't differentiate between what is real and what is a daydream. When you visualise an act, your brain tells your neurons to carry out the act, which creates a new neural pathway that primes your body to perform in a way that is consistent with what you imagined.

\\\\\\\\\\\\\\\\\\\\\\\\\\\\ **EXERCISE** ////////////////////////

1) Go back to the intentions you set for your pregnancy, your birth and when you're a mother and are holding your precious baby in your arms.

2) For each intention, picture yourself as if you're already in that moment and experiencing what you want. Close your eyes. Take in all the tiny details. What do you feel? What can you see? What can you hear? What can you smell?

Don't overthink it—that is engaging the mind. For this exercise you want to engage your senses and visualise them, getting into as much detail as possible.

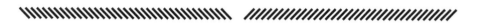

CONCLUSION

I'll never forget my reaction when I first found out I was pregnant. Equal feelings of excitement, fear, disbelief and uncertainty reared to the surface. My life was going to change. My life was going to shift irrevocably whether I was ready or not—soon I would have to leave my specialised IT consulting role to have a baby.

I cried. But not out of joy, out of fear. I wouldn't be footloose and fancy-free and able to have long, lazy, uninterrupted afternoons with my girlfriends. Leland and I couldn't just pop to the movies spontaneously and decide at the end to watch the next film in a marathon movie session of our own making. The goal I'd set to run the Gold Coast Marathon the following year was gone. Like the credits rolling at the end of a movie, the list of what I was going to have to give up scrolled in front of my eyes. I was shell-shocked and so was Leland—except he was shocked at my crazy reaction.

A little while later the shock faded and the realisation set in. I was going to be a mother. I was going to be *a mother*. I was carrying another life. My shock turned into a joyful disbelief. Leland and I would soon shift from being a couple to a being family. The love we have for each other had resulted in creating the life of our child. Our child. Made by us. It was an incredible miracle.

And just as the cliché goes, in that moment, everything changed. I could never be the person I was a few minutes before. The journey to motherhood had begun and so had my quest for knowledge.

That quest culminated in the publication of this book.

I learnt some powerful lessons in my transition to motherhood, and the biggest was a heart opening like I had never experienced. I also learnt that if I can survive (and indeed thrive) in motherhood, I can survive and thrive in anything. It has been an ongoing journey of acceptance and being comfortable with change. Even though I often second-guess myself as a mother, I have come to learn that what my gut feeling and instinct tell me to do is generally the best course of action for our family. I have learnt not to compare myself with others, that the journey our family walks is ours alone, and that I don't always have all the answers. But I have the wonderful support of my partner and our village, and I know we will always get there in the end.

I hope that the knowledge and practical activities in this book will help you find calm in the middle of chaos—like the eye in a storm. Know that you do have the inner strength and resilience to meet whatever comes your way, and that with your heart opening you can stand solid in the highest joys that come with becoming a mother. I trust this book has given you strategies that will let you stand firmly grounded, knowing you are not alone.

RESOURCES AND WHAT'S NEXT

If you would like to dig deeper into any of the strategies unlocked in the book, I invite you to visit my website www.theconnectedmama. com, where you will find materials that support the advice given in this book. You can also sign up to my newsletter which contains valuable information, tips and hints for your transition to motherhood.

With the purchase of It's Your Birth... Right? you also received a complimentary tuition to the 7 Day Connection Challenge (worth $97).

This fun and engaging online challenge supports the knowledge you have gained from this book by having you complete 7 daily, 5-minute exercises.

Please visit www.theconnectedmama.com/7-day-challenge to sign up.

ABOUT THE AUTHOR

A behaviour change specialist and mentor, Cherie Pasion is the founder of Connected Mama.

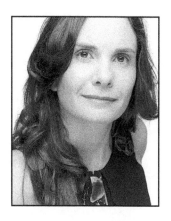

Known for her high-energy and positive outlook, Cherie helps professional women transition calmly from being in their career to motherhood.

In doing so, she draws upon her experience as a mother, Master degree in Social Science and professional background in designing and implementing multiple award-winning behaviour change programs.

Author photo by Portrait Store

Cherie lives in Brisbane, Australia, with her husband and son.

To work with Cherie, have her speak at your event or learn more about her connection compass method and nurturing products, visit:

www.theconnectedmama.com or by email: cherie@theconnectedmama.com

FURTHER RESOURCES

Baby massage
Pinky McKay, *Baby Massage* (DVD)

Breastfeeding
Australian Breastfeeding Association, *Breastfeeding ... naturally* (Book)

Pregnancy and early motherhood nutrition
Gabriela Rosa, *Eat your way to parenthood: The diet secrets of highly fertile couples revealed* (Book) (note, while the main focus is on fertility, the information and recipes are still relevant for pregnancy)

Baby language
Baby Ears by DBL (App)

Baby development
Mayo Clinic, *Mayo Clinic Guide to a Healthy Pregnancy* (Book)

Labour and birth
Cheryl Sheriff, *Stork Talk* (Book)
Janet Balaskas, *Active birth* (Book)
Marie Mongan, *HypnoBirthing: the Marie Mongan style* (Book)
Pam England, *Birthing from Within* (Book)
Toni Harman and Alex Wakefield, *Microbirth Documentary* (DVD)

Miscarriage and loss

Pink Elephants Support Network, www.pinkelephantssupport. com (Website)

Parenting

Stephen Biddulph, *Raising Boys* and *Raising Girls* (Book)

Self care

Kirstie Stockx, *Self Care for New Mums* (Book)

Leonie Percy, *Mother Om* (Book)

Sensory stimulation

Thomas Verny, *The Secret Life of the Unborn Child: How You Can Prepare Your Baby For a Happy, Healthy Life* (Book)

Stress relief

Dr Linda Wilson, *Stress Made Easy: Peeling Women off the Ceiling* (Book)

ENDNOTES

CONNECTIONS ARE AT THE HEART OF MOTHERHOOD

Based on calculator and assumptions provided in 'How many ancestors do you have?' retrieved on 22/01/15 from Family Forest Project http://familyforest.com/resources/51/ancestors-at-a-glance

CONNECT WITH YOU

2   Harman, Bronwyn, (2008) 'The 'Good Mother Syndrome' and Playgroup: The Lived Experience of a Group of Mothers', Doctorate of Psychology thesis, Edith Cowan University, Perth WA, and Marriner, Cosima, 'Motherhood: I thought I could cope with anything' retrieved on 11/10/16 from from The Sydney Morning Herald http://www.smh.com.au/nsw/i-thought-i-could-cope-with-anything-20160715-gq6ebg.html

3   Tolle, Eckhart in interview with Tami Simon, 'The Power of Now and the End of Suffering' retrieved on 25/01/15 from Eckhart Teachings   https://www.eckharttolle.com/article/The-Power-Of-Now-Spirituality-And-The-End-Of-Suffering

4   Chopra, Deepak (2014) '5 Steps for Setting Powerful Intentions' retrieved on 29/01/15 from Chopra Centred Lifestyle http://www.chopra.com/ccl/5-steps-to-setting-powerful-intentions

5   Rodriguez, Tori (2013) 'Negative emotions are the key to wellbeing' retrieved on 25/05/15 from Scientific American http://www.scientificamerican.com/article/negative-emotions-key-wellbeing/?page=1

6   Sarker, P et al (2007) 'Ontegony of foetal exposure to maternal cortisol using midtrimester amniotic fluid as a biomarker', Clinical Endocrinology 66: 636–640. doi:10.1111/j.1365-2265.2007.02785.x

7   Sorgen, Carol (2003) *Bonding with baby before birth*. Retrieved on 07/02/15 from WebMD http://www.webmd.com/baby/features/bonding-with-baby-before-birth

8   Verny, Thomas and Weintraub, Pamela (August 2000) *Nurturing the unborn child: A nine-month program for soothing, stimulating and communicating with your baby*, Kindle edition.

9   Davey, Graham (July 2012) 'The Psychological Effects of TV News' retrieved on 28/05/15 from Pyschology Today https://www.psychologytoday.com/blog/why-we-worry/20twelve06/the-psychological-effects-tv-news

10   Diamond, Terry (2016) 'Emotional Wellbeing, Prioritising Mental Wellness After Pregnancy Loss' retrieved on 20/10/16 from http://pinkelephantssupport.com/wp-content/uploads/2016/10/pinkelephantssupport-emotional-wellbeing-16.pdf

11   Mongan, Marie (2005) *HypnoBirthing The Mongan Method: A natural approach to a safe, easier, more comfortable birthing*, Third edition, Florida:HCI

12   Levett, Kate et al (2016) 'Complementary therapies for labour and birth study: a randomised controlled trial of antenatal integrative medicine for pain management in labour' retrieved on 10/10/2016 from BMJ Open https://bmjopenbeta.bmj.com/content/6/7/e0101691.abstract

13   Information provided by Kathleen Marcoux, Prenatal yoga teacher, Tree of Life Yoga

14   Permission to use exercise provided by Melissa Spilsted, HypnoBirthing Australia

15   Peacock, Fiona (2015) 'Active Birth–8 big benefits for mother and baby' retrieved on 25/07/15 from BellyBelly www.bellybelly.com.au/birth/active-birth/

16   Information provided by Kathleen Marcoux, Prenatal yoga teacher, Tree of Life Yoga

17   Richardson, Nadine (2016), She Births website. Retrieved on 10/10/16 from www.shebirths.com

CONNECT WITH YOUR BABY

18   Verny, Thomas and Weintraub, Pamela (2000) *Nurturing the unborn child: A nine-month program for soothing, stimulating and communicating with your baby*, Kindle edition

19   Verny, Thomas (1982) *The Secret Life of the Unborn Child: How You Can Prepare Your Baby For a Happy, Healthy Life.* New York:Dell

20 Sorgen, Carol (2003) *Bonding with baby before birth.* Retrieved on 07/02/15 from WebMD http://www.webmd.com/baby/features/bonding-with-baby-before-birth

21 Keltner, Dacher (2010) 'Hands on Research: The Science of Truth', Greater Good Science Centre, University of California, Berkeley retrieved on 15/01/15 http://greatergood.berkeley.edu/article/item/hands_on_research

22 Keltner, Dacher (2014) Week 3 course material in The Science of Happiness Course offered by Greater Good Science Centre, University of California, Berkeley on EDx. Retrieved on 14/12/14 http://courses.edx.org

23 McKay, Pinky 'Touch me and help me grow – how massage can make your baby healthier, happier and smarter' retrieved on 26/05/15 from Pinky McKay http://www.pinkymckay.com/touch-me-and-help-me-grow-how-massage-can-boost-your-babys-well-being/

24 '7 Ways to Bond with Your Unborn Baby' retrieved on 12/01/15 from Ask Dr Sears http://www.askdrsears.com/topics/pregnancy-childbirth/fourth-month/7-ways-bond-your-preborn-baby

25 According to research commissioned by Spotify and carried out by Dr Becky Spelman to investigate music that calms the nerves before flying. Retrieved on 20/02/15 from http://www.news.com.au/travel/travel-advice/best-songs-to-listen-to-on-planes-revealed-in-spotify-study/story-e6frfqfr-1226664706235

26 Sorgen, Carol (2003) *Bonding with baby before birth.* Retrieved on 07/02/15 from WebMD http://www.webmd.com/baby/features/bonding-with-baby-before-birth

27   Dewar, Gwen (2009) 'Wired for fast-track learning? The newborn senses of taste and smell' retrieved on 21/7/2015 from http://www.parentingscience.com/newborn-senses.html

28   Dewar, Gwen (2009) 'Flavors in breast milk and baby formula: How early feeding experiences shape your baby's preferences for solid foods' retrieved on 19/7/2015 from Parenting Science http://www.parentingscience.com/flavors-in-breast-milk.html

29   Dewar, Gwen (2009) 'Flavors in breast milk and baby formula: How early feeding experiences shape your baby's preferences for solid foods' retrieved on 19/7/2015 from Parenting Science http://www.parentingscience.com/flavors-in-breast-milk.html; and Dewar, Gwen (2008) 'Nutrients and calories in breast milk: A guide for the science minded' retrieved on 19/7/2015 from Parenting Science http://www.parentingscience.com/calories-in-breast-milk.html

30   Marcobal et al (2010) 'Consumption of Human Milk Oligosaccharides by Gut-related Microbes', Journal of Agricultural and Food Chemistry, 2010 May, 58(9): 5334-5340

31   Tassone, Shawn and Landherr, Kathryn (2014) Spiritual Pregnancy: Develop, Nurture & Embrace the Journey to Motherhood, Minnesota:Lleywellyn Publications

32   University of Montreal, 'Why do you want to eat the baby?' retrieved on 01/06/15 from Universite de Montreal Nouvelle website http://www.nouvelles.umontreal.ca/udem-news/news/20130923-why-do-you-want-to-eat-the-baby.html and Lundstrom Johan et al (2013) 'Maternal status regulates cortical responses to the body odor of newborns' retrieved on 01/06/15 from Frontiers in Psychology

http://journal.frontiersin.org/Journal/10.3389/fpsyg.2013.00597/full

33   Porter and Winberg, (1999) 'Unique salience of maternal breast odors for newborn infants', Neuroscience and Biobehavioural Reviews, 1999;23(3):439-449.

34   Stefano Vaglio, (2009) 'Chemical communication and mother-infant recognition', Communicative & Integrative Biology, 2009 May-Jun; 2(3): 279–281

CONNECT WITH OTHERS

35   Annette Baulch, Relationship coach and founder of OzTantra, www.oztantra.com.au

36   'New baby: preparing your other children' Retrieved on 30/5/15 from Raising Children Network http://raisingchildren.net.au/articles/new_baby_preparing_other_children.html

37   'How to Prepare Your Child for the New Baby' Retrieved on 30/5/15 from Aha Parenting http://www.ahaparenting.com/ages-stages/pregnancy/prepare-your-child-for-new-baby

CONNECT WITH NATURE

38   Russell, Helen et al (2011) 'Pregnancy at work: A national survey', published by the HSE Crisis Pregnancy Programme and the Equality Authority

39   Sarker, P et al (2007) 'Ontegony of foetal exposure to maternal cortisol using midtrimester amniotic fluid as a biomarker', Clinical Endocrinology (Oxf) Volume 66, Issue 5 (May 2007): 636-40

40   Yoshifumi Miyazaki et al (2010) *Trends in research related to 'Shinrin-yoku' (taking in the forest atmosphere or forest bathing) in Japan*, Environmental Health and Preventative Medicine, 2010 Jan;15(1):27-37

41   Silverstone, Matthew (2011) *Blinded by Science*, Kindle edition

42   Wright, Carolanne (2012) 'The incredible benefits of walking barefoot daily' retrieved on 15/02/15 from The Healers Journal http://www.thehealersjournal.com/20twelve/twelve/02/the-incredible-benefits-of-walking-barefoot-daily/

43   Ananda, Kara Maria (2014) 'Therapeutic Benefits of Water for Pregnancy, Birth and Babies' retrieved on 20/2/15 from http://karamariaananda.com/blog/2013/12/1/the-healing-benefits-of-water-for-pregnancy-labor-birth; Bolitho and Hatch (2014) *Aqua Exercise for pregnancy and postnatal health* (London:Bloomsbury)

44   Royal Brisbane and Women's Hospital Women's and Newborn Services (2012) *Birth Centre Handbook.*

45   Yoshifumi Miyazaki et al (2010) *Trends in research related to 'Shinrin-yoku' (taking in the forest atmosphere or forest bathing) in Japan*, Environmental Health and Preventative Medicine, 2010 Jan;15(1):27-37

46   Lipman, Frank (2013) 'Get out there: Nature's Healing Power' retrieved on 06/02/15 from http://www.drfranklipman.com/get-out-there/

47   Environmental Working Group, '2015 Shopper's Guide to Pesticides in Produce' retrieved on 31/05/15 from http://www.ewg.org/foodnews/

48   National Institute of Environmental Health Sciences, 'Endocrine Disruptors', retrieved on 30/05/15 from www.niehs.nih.gov

MAINTAINING CONNECTIONS

49   Thomas Verny (1982) *The Secret Life of the Unborn Child: How You Can Prepare Your Baby For a Happy, Healthy Life*. New York: Dell

50   Olga Kabel, 'Yogis ahead of science: One nostril breathing determines how you feel' retrieved on 31/05/15 fromwww.sequencewiz.org; Stancak and Kuna, (1994)'EEG changes during forced alternate nostril breathing', International Journal of Psychophysiology, October 1994, Vol 18(1): 75-79

51   Emmons, Robert (2010) 'Why Gratitude is Good' retrieved on 25/7/15 from Greater Good Science Centre, Berkeley University of California http://greatergood.berkeley.edu/article/item/why_gratitude_is_good

52   Philip Watkins, *Gratitude and the good life: Towards a Psychology of Appreciation* eBook version.

53   U.S. Pranic Healing Centre, 'What is Pranic Healing?' retrieved on 04/11/15 from http://pranichealing.com/what-pranic-healing

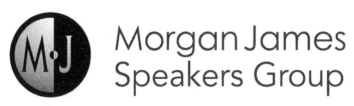

Morgan James
Speakers Group

We connect Morgan James published
authors with live and online events
and audiences whom will benefit
from their expertise.

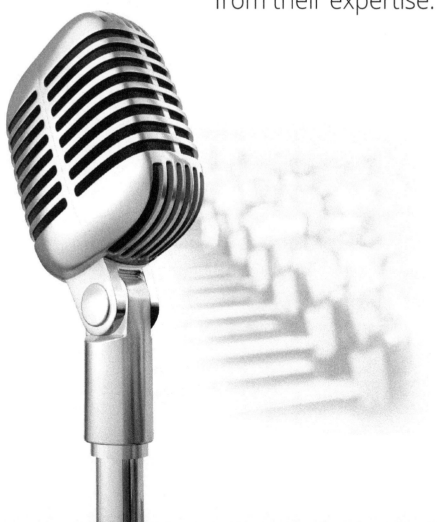

 Morgan James makes all of our titles available
through the Library for All Charity Organization.

www.LibraryForAll.org